RUNNING WITHOUT FEAR

Other books by Kenneth H. Cooper, M.D.

AEROBICS

THE NEW AEROBICS

AEROBICS FOR WOMEN
(with Mildred Cooper)

THE AEROBICS WAY

THE AEROBICS PROGRAM FOR TOTAL WELL-BEING

RUNNING WITHOUT FEAR

How to Reduce the Risk of Heart Attack and Sudden Death During Aerobic Exercise

Kenneth H. Cooper, M.D., M.P.H.

M. Evans and Company, Inc.
NEW YORK

This book does not substitute for the medical advice and supervision of your personal physician. No medical therapy or exercise program should be undertaken except under the direction of a physician.

Library of Congress Cataloging in Publication Data

Cooper, Kenneth H.
  Running without fear.

  Bibliography: p.
  Includes index.
    1. Heart—Infarction—Prevention. 2. Sudden death—
Prevention. 3. Running—Physiological aspects.
4. Exercise tests. 5. Aerobic exercises. I. Title.
RC685.I6C66   1985   616.1'23705   85–4501

ISBN 0-87131-456-8

M. Evans and Company, Inc.
216 East 49 Street
New York, New York 10017

Design by Ronald F. Shey

Manufactured in the United States of America

9 8 7 6 5 4 3 2 1

To the millions of people who are exercising regularly in their pursuit of good health. May this book allay any fears they might have and give them reassurance that what they are doing is right.

CONTENTS

PREFACE

On July 21, 1984, I was on a weekend outing with my family at a lake near Dallas. While the children were swimming, my wife and I were relaxing on the beach. But I was disturbed that a portable radio nearby was disrupting my nap—until I heard, "Jim Fixx, the author of *The Complete Book of Running* dies while jogging!"

Having been only partially awake, I wasn't sure what I had heard. I asked my wife, Millie, "Did you hear that?"

"No," she replied. And when I told her, she said, "You must have made a mistake. We were with Jim just a short time ago."

Soon, I discovered that the radio announcer had said exactly what I thought. But little did I realize the impact Jim's death would have on my life and on joggers and runners all over the world. The press, the media, Jim's followers, nonexercisers, and the merely curious came to me or called from everywhere and they all asked the same question: "How could Jim Fixx die while jogging?"

I was convinced that someone in a knowledgeable position had to allay apprehension and respond to those inquiries or the whole exercise movement of the past fifteen years would be in jeopardy. Substantiating my concern were articles published with such titles as "Fitness Boom to Go Into Decline in Response to Fixx's Death." So immediately, I initiated a thorough study to ascertain the events surrounding Jim's death, the results of the autopsy, and the existence of any medical problems that could have contributed to his death.

In addition, I tried to obtain answers to the question: What do we really know about exercise and its relationship to heart attacks?

To determine in detail the events surrounding Jim's death, I enlisted the assistance of a friend, William Proctor, who is not only an author, a graduate of Harvard Law School, and a qualified attorney, but also a former New York newspaper reporter. Proctor traveled to Hardwick, Vermont, stayed at the motel where Jim had spent his final hours, and conducted an on-site inspection of the route over which Jim made his final run.

During his time in Vermont, Proctor had in-depth interviews with the police, motel personnel, and State medical officials who were knowledgeable about the case. In addition to his research in Vermont, Proctor conducted interviews with family members and others who knew the most about Jim's life and death. I had the privilege of becoming personally acquainted with Jim's son John, who was most helpful and cooperative in every way, and particularly in obtaining all available medical records.

Finally, Proctor combed through library sources and other records to compile what has become the most complete report on the events preceding and following Jim Fixx's death. The events and dialogue presented in the following pages are based directly on this exhaustive investigation.

In attempting to answer the question—the relationship between exercise and heart attacks—I have carefully evaluated the research coming from our own Institute for Aerobics Research. I have also studied the current exercise and cardiology literature, particularly that which was published after 1980. This analysis of the literature has become even more important in view of recent publications highly critical of the value of exercise.

I would ask that the reader look objectively at the information contained in this book, analyze it, and then reach an independent conclusion. I believe you will discover, as I did, that there were factors other than coronary artery disease that may have played a role in Jim's death. Also, it seems clear that the current literature documenting the value of exercise in maintaining good health and preventing disease is far too impressive to be ignored.

If my goals in writing this book are achieved, those of you who are exercising will be remotivated; those who are not exercising will seriously question the wisdom of that decision; and by adhering to the guidelines outlined in the following pages, people will once again be able to run, cycle, swim, and dance aerobically—without fear! Finally, may you discover that exercise is not the only key to health and longevity, but that it is the means by which life can be enjoyed to the fullest.

ACKNOWLEDGMENTS

To list all the people who in some way helped in the preparation of this book would be an impossibility. Yet I would be remiss not to recognize a few special contributions. William Proctor was outstanding in his investigative reporting of the details surrounding the death of Jim Fixx; in addition, he provided great assistance in the preparation of the final manuscript. Lewis Calver was the artist responsible for all the detailed drawings in the book, and my very competent assistant, Harold Burkhalter, worked many hours reviewing patients' charts, compiling data, and screening journal articles. Dr. Larry Gibbons, director of the Cooper Clinic, was one of the reviewers of the book and also provided the recommendations for the frequency of exercise testing as found in the Appendix. Dr. Steven Blair, director of epidemiology for the Institute for Aerobics Research, reviewed the book and made very important suggestions and recommendations. Dr. Eleanor McQuillen, chief medical examiner for the state of Vermont, was most helpful in providing the details of James Fixx's autopsy. Several members of the Fixx family provided assistance, but Kitty Fixx Bower and John Fixx were especially supportive and most generous in giving of their time. My secretary, Harriet Guthrie, continues to amaze me with her organizational ability, which was so critical in enabling me to handle all my other responsibilities in addition to those associated with the preparation of this book. And finally, a special word of thanks is due to my wife, Millie; my daughter, Berkley; and my son, Tyler; who always support me unquestioningly in my multiple endeavors.

CHAPTER ONE

THE JIM FIXX SYNDROME: WHAT IT IS AND HOW TO PREVENT IT

Exercise is absolutely essential to good health. It's the cornerstone for any complete effort to reduce the risk of heart attack and sudden death. It's also a major key to an energetic, long life.

Yet, today, exercise is under attack. It's the needless victim of distortion and misunderstanding. In this book, I want to clear away the confusion and try to set the record straight. Above all, I want to provide you with solid grounds to feel totally confident as you fit aerobic exercise into your own approach to good health and longer life.

The role of exercise in a complete health maintenance program has become so obvious that few reputable scientists and physicians today would argue with its importance. Indeed, one of the most recent issues of the prestigious *New England Journal of Medicine* reported that those who engage regularly in vigorous exercise, such as jogging, *definitely* reduce their overall risk of sudden death from a heart attack.

But despite such evidence, the precise role that exercise should play isn't always clearly understood, even by the medical establishment. On one hand, there are still a few vocal critics who, despite the evidence, try to argue that endurance workouts are clearly dangerous. They say regular, vigorous exercise, even when pursued by the most exacting safety standards, is conducive to sudden death, and therefore should be avoided. These naysayers found fuel for their attacks in the tragic death of the best-selling author James Fixx, who had become one of the most visible and effective evangelists for aerobic exercise.

On the other hand, there are those who believe that a regimen of long-distance running, swimming, or cycling will solve all ills and wipe out any possibility of heart disease. They have become victims of a syndrome that raises exercise to an undeserved level of super-panacea. We'll explore this mind-set in some detail in just a moment.

In any case, what we face today is widespread confusion and ignorance about exactly what exercise can or can't do. So, in the following pages I want to show you how you can continue to run, swim, cycle, or dance, and get the maximum health benefits of that aerobic activity—*without fear*. At the same time, you'll be able to reduce your risk of a heart attack or sudden death, both when you're exercising *and* when you're pursuing any of your other, less strenuous, daily activities.

To understand the approach to physical activity that can provide you with the greatest health benefits, it's always helpful to focus first on a concrete case study. So now, let's consider the implications of one of the most tragic and widely reported events in the recent history of preventive medicine—the death of a man who was already on his way to becoming a legend in the annals of aerobic exercise.

At special times and places, historical events converge to produce a personality who rises to the heights, to a realm of celebrity and influence reaching far beyond the ordinary. Often, this individual becomes a standard-bearer of major movements already afoot; he may also become a symbol of great ideals yet to be realized.

His name becomes virtually indistinguishable from the cause he espouses; his word can motivate his followers to feats they had previously regarded as above their capacities. His mere presence may actually inspire the uncommitted to affirm an entirely new way of life. History, in short, sometimes gives birth to a hero.

In his own way, James F. Fixx was such a man. For a time, his name became virtually synonymous with running. His writings inspired untold thousands to change their lives and aspire to new heights of health and energetic living.

Specifically, Jim Fixx emerged onto the national and international scene in October 1977 with the incredible bestseller, *The Complete Book of Running*. The book hit the *New York Times* bestseller list by the end of November 1977 and soon rose to the number one position. It finally dropped off the list nearly two years later, but only after setting all sorts of records for hardcover publishing.

By then, the name "Jim Fixx" had become a household word. His muscular legs, which adorned the striking covers of his books, became as familiar to some segments of the public as the logos of the world's largest corporations. He was well on his way to becoming a legend in his own time, with more than a million readers and probably as many jogging enthusiasts who hung on his every word. Nor was Fixx's celebrity a hollow sort of notoriety. Through his fame he helped promote important ideas that enhanced public health.

It happened this way: His book rose to the top of the bestseller charts in the midst of a major surge of interest in the benefits of exercise and an unprecedented decline in deaths from heart disease. According to the Gallup Poll, 24 percent of adult Americans were exercising regularly in 1961, and that number had risen to 47 percent by 1977, the year *The Complete Book of Running* was published. By 1984, the figure was up to 59 percent—an increase that must, at least in part, be attributed to the Fixx inspiration.

At the same time that exercise was increasing, heart deaths were decreasing. There were 511.6 deaths from cardiovascular diseases per 100,000 population in 1961, according to the National Center for Health Statistics. That number dropped to 437.5 in 1977, and finally to 424.2 in 1981, the last date when such figures are available.

So Jim Fixx emerged as the exercise boom was on the upsurge, and he spurred it on to even greater heights. But most heroes have a day of reckoning, and Jim Fixx's final hour was one of the most devastating imaginable, in light of what he had come to symbolize.

On July 20, 1984, on a rural roadside in Vermont, this internationally known advocate of aerobic exercise, though only fifty-two years of age, collapsed and died during one of his daily runs. He had fallen victim to the very heart disease he had tried to help so many to escape.

It seemed that the Fates had conspired to commit the supreme irony, with the runner's runner succumbing at the hand of the very activity he had lived for so successfully and energetically. Also, a wave of fear swelled up in the wake of the Fixx tragedy. To much of the public, it appeared that exercise might be a two-edged sword, with perhaps more perils than benefits.

I myself was shocked and dismayed by the untimely death of Jim, whom I had come to regard as a friend and colleague. But soon, my personal sadness widened into a deeper concern for the future of the entire preventive medicine and exercise movements. People are living more energetically these days, and they are also living longer because of the motivational ability of leaders like Jim Fixx. Yet the irony of his death at a relatively young age spurred some negative thinkers and sedentary scientists to hop onto an anti-exercise bandwagon.

My phone literally rang off the hook for weeks after Jim's death, as I was bombarded by both the media and medical establishment with questions about the meaning of the event. I still find that queries about the Fixx death preoccupy significant segments of audiences during my lectures.

Popular publications became obsessed with the subject. Headlines in newspapers, such as one that screamed "Fixx's Death May Slow the Fitness Boom," fed the growing hysteria. Then, author James Michener, in a major article entitled "Living with an Ailing Heart" in *The New York Times Magazine* (August 19, 1984), led off with these words:

"The dramatic death of James F. Fixx, guru of exercise fanatics, of whom I am one, has thrown a scare into the jogging fraternity. How could a youngish man, who exercised regularly and preached the benefits of a sane life, go out for an afternoon run along a country road in Vermont and drop dead? The case was a real shocker. . . ."

Yes, it was indeed a shocker. And the way various writers and exercise enthusiasts have voiced their worries can be quite revealing. Their expressions of dismay at Fixx's death frequently reflect some prevalent but entirely false assumptions.

During the euphoria of the recent fitness boom, many people began to believe that exercise could render an individual virtually invulnerable to sudden death, and especially to death from heart-related problems. Exercise thus became the long sought-after elixir of long life.

Jim Fixx himself may have bought these assumptions to one extent or another. But there's an even more important consideration than what Fixx himself believed. The big difficulty is that a webwork of mistaken beliefs about exercise has become an integral part of the thinking of many people who identify with Fixx and his philosophy of good health. Consequently, I've chosen the term "Jim Fixx Syndrome" to describe those who, in one way or another, accept exercise as the ultimate antidote to heart disease and sudden death.

In medical parlance, a syndrome is a group of symptoms and physical signals which, when they appear in one person at the same time, form the pattern for a certain illness or abnormal condition. So, the Jim Fixx Syndrome involves an abnormal belief that an aerobic exerciser is more or less impervious to coronary illness. Also, the Syndrome usually involves one or more of four clearly identifiable "myths of invulnerability."

Before we get into a more detailed discussion of these myths, however, I should mention one qualification to much of what I'll be saying throughout this book. Because Jim Fixx was a runner, a lot of my observations and advice will be addressed to runners. But as you'll see as we progress through the discussion of sudden death, stress tests, and other topics, all of these points about the impact of exercise on your body apply to other forms of aerobic exercise as well.

So, if you're a swimmer, cross-country skier, squash player, cycler, aerobic dancer, or walker, just keep this in mind: the myths of invulnerability which make up the Jim Fixx Syndrome apply to you as much as to your colleague who is jogging along down the nearest highway.

Now, let's examine each of the myths of invulnerability about exercise and explore what it may mean to you personally and to your fitness program.

Myth #1: I Couldn't Have Heart Disease and Run the Way I Run Without Symptoms

I can hardly count the number of runners, swimmers, cyclists, and other aerobic exercisers I've met who hold this belief.

Jim Fixx himself, in his *Second Book of Running*, said, "Heart attacks, while not unknown in trained runners, are so rare as to be of negligible probability." Then, he went on to quote approvingly a doctor who declared, "The only thing that can kill a healthy runner, other than cars and buses, is heat stroke."

According to several reports, Fixx regularly ran 60 to 70 miles a week for at least twelve years. By my calculations, he must have logged in more than 37,000 miles during his career. That represents a lot of road and a lot of running shoe rubber.

But more than the quantity of mileage, there are some important assumptions that underlie this level of dedication. There is often a conviction that if you start running or doing other distance exercise beyond a certain quasi-magical period of time, you somehow become invulnerable. In effect, you acquire a guarantee that you won't develop coronary problems. Supposedly, you move into a realm of fitness that allows you to transcend all heart attacks and hardening of the arteries (arteriosclerosis).

Nothing could be further from the truth. There is absolutely nothing known to man that is totally protective against coronary heart disease, whether it is medicine, surgery, or marathon running.

Furthermore, the heart is masterful at disguising its problems. You can run along for miles and miles at a heart rate of 150 or 160 beats per minute. You may feel quite energetic, and you certainly may not experience any pain. But even as you run, you could be suffering from serious clogging (occlusion) of the arteries leading to the heart. In fact, sudden death may lurk just around the corner unless you take steps, other than exercise, to correct your condition.

The possible existence of such serious coronary artery disease is the reason that I emphasize the importance of regular, expert treadmill stress testing *at or near maximum,* particularly if you are past forty years of age. This test is especially important if you're in the habit of "kicking in," or sprinting, at the end of exercise.

In a recently published article, Dr. Larry Gibbons, who is on our staff at the Aerobics Center in Dallas, studied a group of subjects who had abnormal exercise tests. Some abnormalities occurred prior to 85 percent of predicted maximum heart rates; some occurred only as the subjects approached maximum exertion. During the study, Gibbons discovered a disturbing phenomenon: 39 percent of those with abnormal stress electrocardiograms escaped detection at the 85-percent level, simply because they were *not* pushed to their maximum effort and heart rate. No angina (chest pain) and no abnormal readings showed on their electrocardiograms at the lower heart rate. It was only at close to 100 percent of maximum performance that abnormalities were detected.

Now, let's apply these findings to your personal situation: Suppose you are exercising at 135 beats per minute as in the above example, and your maximum heart rate is 185. In this case, you would be working out at only 73 percent of your maximum capacity. Then, you execute a "kick" or sprint at the end of your run, so that your heart rate rises up to or close to the maximum 185 beats per minute. If you're suffering from undiagnosed coronary artery disease, such strain could cause serious problems . . . even though you may never have experienced any prior warning signals like chest pain. Only a properly conducted stress test has the capacity to reveal the serious heart problems that could occur at maximal levels of exercise.

Clearly, then, you can run the way you run, or swim the way you swim, or cycle the way you cycle without *any* symptoms—and *still* have heart disease.

Myth #2: People Who Run Marathons Don't Die of Heart Attacks

This myth of invulnerability is peculiar to highly trained long-distance runners. Some people actually used to think that just training for and running a marathon would automatically eliminate the possibility of heart disease. Of course, this notion just involves carrying the first myth to its logical conclusion. In other words, if running long distances protects you from heart disease, then running *very* long distances must be even better.

When studies started appearing on marathoners who had died of heart disease, the absurdity of this belief became apparent. One of the most recent I'm aware of was conducted by Dr. Thomas Bassler, a California pathologist. He reported in a letter in the July 27, 1984 issue of the *Journal of the American Medical Association,* an investigation into why some fourteen marathoners had died of cardiovascular disease. His conclusion: Inadequate nutrition had contributed to their deaths.

Ironically, Bassler at one time gained notoriety as a major proponent of the notion that anyone who finished a marathon in less than four hours was immune to heart disease. While Jim Fixx didn't give

Bassler's ideas an outright endorsement, he did refer to his work approvingly on at least one occasion: "Although not all of Bassler's medical colleagues agree with him [about marathon immunity], he does have a wide following" (*The Complete Book of Running*).

Of course, the idea that running a marathon provides some sort of invulnerability to heart disease is sheer nonsense. Fixx recognized the weaknesses in that argument in his later writings. But there are still many uninformed runners, swimmers, and other aerobic exercisers who fall into this trap. They believe that training for and then running a marathon or some equivalent maximum distance in another sport in a respectable time provides a seal against the onslaught of coronary artery problems.

What this mistaken notion overlooks is that other factors, such as poor diet or heredity, may be undoing all the benefits an individual is achieving by running. As I said in my previous book, *The Aerobics Program for Total Well-Being*, if you're running more than 12 to 15 miles per week, you're running for reasons other than cardiovascular health. For example, you may be running to condition yourself for competitive racing. Or you may be running because you have a "positive addiction" to the sport. Or you may be running because the activity provides a social outlet with other long-distance enthusiasts.

But those are not reasons related to good health. For complete cardiovascular fitness, all you need to run is 12 to 15 miles a week.

Such moderate distances, when combined with a low-fat diet, no smoking, regular comprehensive medical check-ups, and other ingredients of a healthy lifestyle, provide as much protection against heart disease as you can get. And even then, there can be no absolute guarantee that a family history of heart disease or some other factor may not prevail.

Myth #3: Stress Tests Are Worthless Because They Produce Too Many False Readings (False Positives and Negatives). Also, Physicians Don't Know How to Interpret the Stress Electrocardiogram of an Athlete

Although Jim Fixx had at least one stress test, he apparently subscribed to the belief that they are more or less useless. His former wife, Alice, had been urging him to get a complete physical, and he told her that he would check with a physician friend and abide by his advice.

He was told: "Annual physicals are a waste of time. For runners, they're even dangerous. You're likely to run into a doctor who doesn't like your electrocardiogram, and before you know it you'll be in the Mayo Clinic having coronary-artery studies. . . . Stress tests . . . are virtually useless in athletes—and they're not always very useful for other people" (*The Complete Book of Running*).

The physician did moderate his remarks by saying, "Still, if you can find a doctor who won't be stampeded, I do think it's valuable to have tests we can compare later if anything goes wrong."

But even with this qualification, there seems to be a definite bias here against the validity of stress testing—a bias that Jim Fixx apparently accepted too. In fact, he visited the Aerobics Center six months before his death to write a story on Johnny Kelley, the longtime Boston Marathoner. I invited Jim to undergo a stress test, but he declined. Johnny agreed to try the treadmill stress test and did quite well on it. But Jim opted to sit on the sidelines for reasons known only to him.

Jim's sister, Kitty Fixx Bower, later told me that Jim was suffering from a respiratory ailment during his stay in Dallas and that he was probably concerned that he might not perform as well as he might if he were completely well. She feels that he wasn't opposed to the idea of taking a stress test.

Unfortunately, if Jim Fixx had chosen to be tested, there is a very good chance that we would have noticed his coronary artery disease during the examination. Then, we could have prescribed treatment that might well have saved his life.

We'll be going into the question of stress testing in great detail in later chapters. For now, though, let me just say that the criticisms of the accuracy of treadmill stress tests are usually directed against those tests which are inadequately conducted. Many of the studies that attack stress testing generally actually apply only to the so-called "bipolar" system, which requires only three electrodes (rubber patches with wires leading to an electrocardiograph) on the upper body.

What the critics often don't recognize is that as you increase the number of electrodes and "leads" (or electrical fields), the sensitivity and accuracy of the test increases. For an adequate test, you need *at least* seven electrodes on the chest; this provides a nine-lead monitoring system. It's also necessary that you be pushed to a level of exercise that raises your heart rate to its maximum level.

At the Aerobics Center, we always do maximum-performance testing, and we use a fourteen-electrode, fifteen-lead system. This gives us a high degree of accuracy in our testing. In fact, when our method is compared to coronary arteriography, we approach 80-percent "sensitivity," or true readings, in the tests we perform.

Another important factor is the expertise of the technician or physician administering the test. If you are undergoing a test that's being supervised by someone who lacks experience, then the chances increase that you'll get false readings. So it's not the stress test that causes the problems. It's the way the stress test is conducted.

Myth #4: If You Are a Highly Conditioned Long-Distance Runner, You Can Forget Your Heredity

It has become increasingly apparent that one of the most dangerous and decisive risk factors in the development of heart disease is a poor family history. In other words, if your mother or father, or your paternal or maternal grandparents, died of a heart-related cause before age sixty, and especially before age fifty, your chances of dying of the same problem greatly increase. I believe it was the late Dr. Paul Dudley White, a renowned physician, who once said, "If you want to protect yourself from having a heart attack, you must select the proper parents!"

Of course, there is no way you can completely wipe out this risk factor. You can't simply wish away your heredity, any more than you can wish away the two packs of cigarettes a day that you may be smoking.

It *is* true that you can take certain steps which reduce the impact of the heredity factor. For example, if you are smoking two packs a day, you can quit. Or you can drastically reduce the amount of fats and cholesterol in your diet. Or you can embark on a regular aerobic exercise program.

But even as you take these constructive steps, it's important not to fall prey to the prevalent trap of wishful thinking. For example, some people become so convinced of the tremendous benefits of exercise that they eventually convince themselves that exercise by itself is an absolute antidote to heredity.

This attitude may have been something of a temptation for Jim Fixx. As you may know, Jim's father died of a heart attack at the very young age of forty-three, and that tragedy always loomed rather large in his mind.

In his most evenhanded moments, he acknowledged that of all the risk factors related to heart attacks, "exercise may improve all except heredity" (*The Complete Book of Running*).

At the same time, there are indications in his writings that he may have begun to regard exercise as some sort of panacea that could overcome his family history. For one thing, he tended to emphasize exercise to the exclusion of other important preventive health measures, such as the regular preventive medical exam. Also, his writings sounded a hopeful note about the way exercise might swing the pendulum away from heredity: "Running can therefore significantly reduce the risk of developing coronary heart disease, a fact that has long impressed me, since my own coronary heredity is not all it might be" (*Complete*).

Later, his views became even more optimistic about the prospects for exercise. In citing the evidence for the benefits of regular aerobic workouts, he wrote, "As the numbers piled up, the evidence grew that exercise could to some extent overcome every known risk factor, both separately and in all possible combinations. . . . Exercise could reduce, and in some cases nullify, the effects of everything from diabetes to family history" (*Second*).

The essence of this fourth myth is that exercise can do it all. And that, of course, is all wrong. True, exercise may help mitigate the impact of bad heredity. But the background of blood relationships will always be there, and this risk factor may be so powerful in some individuals that ordinary preventive measures will fall short.

Some people have such a strong genetic predisposition to develop coronary disease that they have in effect been *stamped* with that problem. I can prescribe exercise, weight loss, dietary change, and a variety of other "natural" measures. But none of these steps may help. The only answer may be to prescribe medications to control a bad lipid (fat) profile in the blood. Or I may have to recommend bypass surgery.

But these are the extreme cases. For most people with a poor family history of heart disease, a completely natural preventive health program may help immeasurably. Such an approach will certainly include aerobic exercise. But just as important will be the elimination of cigarette smoking, a change in diet, the adoption of a less stressful lifestyle, a loss of weight, regular medical examinations with stress tests, and other features.

These, then, are the four "myths of invulnerability" that make up the Jim Fixx Syndrome. Being misled by just one of them is enough to get you into hot water. As a matter of fact, believing and following only one may be enough to kill you.

But if you can shake free of these myths, you'll be in a better position to understand how exercise can be an indispensable part of a proper preventive health program.

My purpose in the following pages is to give you the facts, not the fantasies about exercise. To this end, we'll explore such issues as:

- What probably killed Jim Fixx, and what can we learn from his tragic death?
- How, when, and where is sudden death most likely to strike?
- What are the eleven "Rules of Risk" for developing heart disease—and how can you reduce them?
- Why is the "cool-down" phase of exercise the most dangerous, and how can you get through it safely?
- What are some safe strategies for specific exercise programs?
- What constitutes an effective stress test, and why is this procedure an important key to good health?
- What exactly is the new Cooper Protocol, the latest, state-of-the-art procedure in stress testing that we've developed at the Institute for Aerobics Research in Dallas?
- Can you really prolong your life?

Let's embark on an exploration of some extremely important but poorly understood facts about that proven elixir of well-being, aerobic exercise. When properly understood, this cornerstone of physical well-being can help you reduce your risk of heart disease, improve the quality of your health, and perhaps even prolong your life.

The first stop on our journey is a rural road just outside a tiny village in northern Vermont.

CHAPTER TWO

WHY DID JIM FIXX DIE?

Jim Fixx was exhausted. It had been a long, hot drive from Cape Cod to the tiny Vermont town of Hardwick—about seven hours with the Friday traffic—and he was hungry and tired. He typically ate very little before his evening meal, and today, July 20, 1984, was no exception. So, as he pulled his Volvo station wagon into the Village Motel at 4:30 P.M., Jim had only two things on his mind: rest and food.

He would soon be moving into a rented Vermont summer house on nearby Caspian Lake, where he planned to finish work on his next book, a thoroughly researched report on sports performance. Northern Vermont was definitely out of the mainstream of the publishing world, but Jim felt comfortable being alone.

In fact, he actually hated the strain and pressure of public life. The constant round of interviews and promotion tours that his books had required of him in recent years produced more pain than inner peace. His body and emotions didn't take well to notoriety. He had even suffered a series of anxiety attacks after a particularly heavy dose of television and radio talk shows a few years back.

The dizziness had stopped, but the stress was as bad as ever. At least, that's what he had been recording in his diary in recent months. For Jim, success seemed to beget stress, and stress was something he needed to avoid if he hoped to function most effectively.

Jim worked best when he was off in a quiet, secluded spot by himself. In fact, he valued his privacy so much that in 1977 he had quit a career in the pressure-packed world of New York City magazine publishing and had gone into the relatively solitary and self-directed world of freelance writing. And he had flourished in this environment. In the solitude of his study in Connecticut, he had turned out *The Complete Book of Running*.

So it was natural he would have headed for an out-of-the-way spot in Vermont to continue his work. He wouldn't be doing any writing in Hardwick, however. That was just a place with a soft bed and a few square meals, a temporary stopover until he could make final arrangements for his lakeside house.

When he walked up to the motel registration desk, the clerk on duty, Patty Dickson, thought he looked like he'd had a hard day. Especially around the eyes: they were lackluster and bloodshot. He appeared to her to be a guy who should just take a shower and go to bed.

"I want a quiet room, away from everybody else," Jim said.

"You can have Room 12—that's on the end," Patty replied as she handed him a registration form.

"I don't feel like unpacking all that stuff out in my car, either," Jim said. "Will it be okay if I leave it there?"

"Nobody will touch it," Patty assured him.

Food was the other thing on Jim's mind. "How about the restaurants around here? Where can I get some good food and a beer with my dinner? A place where it's kind of cool and I can relax."

"You could try Mary Lou's."

The way this man looked, Patty expected him to go directly out for supper and then hit the sack early that night. But that wasn't Jim. Regardless of how tired he might be, he always put on his running shoes and hit the road. Usually for ten miles at a shot. Ten miles a day, seven days a week. That was Jim's style, his commitment, as it had been for more than a decade. Ten miles a day, seven days and seventy miles a week.

But today the conditions were too hot and too hilly. Nearly eighty degrees on this partly cloudy, still, summer afternoon. Perhaps a little disappointing for anyone who expects northern Vermont always to harbor some cool mountain breezes, even in July.

Jim Fixx wasn't in the habit of letting weather interfere with his seven-day-a-week running regimen, however. So the first thing he did, after he went into Room 12, was to strip off his blue tee-shirt and place his wallet on the table. Then, wearing only his blue, white-striped jogging shorts, Nike running shoes, and a stopwatch, he walked right back outside into the heat. He put his room key over his left front tire. That way, he could keep his room locked and still avoid carrying the key during his run.

It was about 4:40 P.M. when Jim started his jog eastward on Route 15. As was his custom, he ran against traffic, on the narrow left shoulder of the road. But there really wasn't much traffic. There rarely is on the roads that run through the farming country in that part of Vermont.

The countryside offered some pleasant, restful scenes: a brook down below him to his left and clumps of trees alternating with rolling farmland as he gazed farther into the distance. It was the kind of landscape that could make a runner glad to be alive on the right kind of day.

But this day wasn't quite like any other. The air remained calm and hot, and the terrain Jim had chosen for his daily jog had a series of steep inclines. When he passed a Chrysler garage only about a half mile from the motel, he was already perspiring heavily. Still, he was moving along steadily, and to a woman at an office in the garage who noticed him, there didn't seem to be anything unusual or memorable about him—except perhaps for the fact that he was a jogger. In that part of the country, you don't see too many joggers on rural highways and back roads.

But then, something apparently started to go wrong. Perhaps it was the rugged country road or the heat, which wouldn't let up. In fact, the temperature began to rise a degree or so as the late afternoon sun broke through the clouds. Or maybe it was Jim's growing fatigue, from his lack of food on top of a grueling six- to seven-hour drive.

Whatever the cause, Jim did something he rarely did: He decided to cut short his daily ten-mile run. This day, he would settle for only about four miles, and a relatively slow four at that. He had run several marathons at a pace of about seven-and-a-half minutes per mile. It would be hard for anyone fifty-two years old, even an athlete as well-conditioned as Jim Fixx, to do much better than nine or ten minutes a mile over this Vermont terrain.

So, somewhere around Route 16, which cuts into Route 15 from the north, exactly two miles from the Village Motel, he turned back. We can only speculate about what he may have been thinking or feeling during this return leg of his run. It wasn't an easy effort because there were still as many "ups" as "downs" on the way back. When a runner, even an experienced one, is working fairly hard over tough terrain to finish a workout, it's difficult to think of anything but the rhythmic pounding of feet, and the road. Always, the road.

Sometimes, though, another thought may stick in the mind, like a kind of aerobically imposed meditation. Jim's thoughts may have settled on his friend Peggy Palmer, or his sister Kitty, or his brother-in-law Jim Bower, all of whom he had left behind when he drove away from Cape Cod that morning. Maybe he was musing about that final scene, when he and Bower were clowning around for a snapshot in front of his packed-up Volvo.

More likely, though, his mind was riveted to the road. The unforgiving road, and the uncomfortable heat. When the Village Motel came into sight, he may have felt some relief. A cold shower, an air-conditioned restaurant, and a cold beer lay just minutes away.

Then, for some reason, he stopped next to a steep, grassy hill that rose from the very edge of Route 15, just across the street from the graded driveway leading down to the motel. He was only about forty or fifty yards from the front door to his room, number 12. Perhaps he halted to check his pulse rate. Or perhaps he wanted one last look at the brook that followed the course of the road. Or perhaps he was already in trouble when he stopped.

Whatever the reason, there is strong evidence that he did stop. And that was when the brief blast of pain, or perhaps just an overpowering feeling of weight, hit him like a Mack truck in his chest. His knees buckled, and he crumpled to the ground, with his left side pressing against the steep hill that jutted out almost into the road. He was found on his knees, with his upper body nearly upright, slumped against the soft grass of the sharply rising slope.

Thus ended the life and the last run of one of the greatest contemporary heroes of endurance exercise.

Why did Jim Fixx die? That's a question that has worried many, from medical authorities and competitive athletes, to middle-aged exercisers. Most amateur exercisers run, swim or cycle just to keep fit and, they hope, to ward off life-threatening illness. But now, with their hero mysteriously dead, they may find themselves wondering, "Is this running (swimming . . . cycling) really good for me? Or is it just another form of Russian roulette? Could I be setting myself up like Jim Fixx for some sort of sudden death? What really happened to Jim Fixx?"

Yes, what *did* happen to Fixx? That's the first key question as we begin to explore how to exercise safely, with the maximum health benefits and the minimum chance of sudden death.

If Fixx's death represents some common danger of endurance exercise, then all of us who work out regularly may be in big trouble. On the other hand, if he died from some special, unique causes, the rest of us may not have so much to worry about. Also, if we can identify anything he may have done wrong, perhaps we can learn some lessons that may help us reduce our personal risk of sudden death and heart disease. So now, let's take a closer look at the man Jim Fixx and attempt to unravel the mystery surrounding his death.

First of all, what do we know about his health history?

When you are alive, you're ignorant about much of what's going on inside your body. Perhaps your lungs, your liver, your arteries, and your heart are just fine. But then again, perhaps they're not. Current medical testing practices for the person without symptoms can tell us a great deal. Unfortunately, however, it takes a complete autopsy to reveal the exact condition of our bodies. So, of course, that means only the dead can tell the full tale about their own bodies.

Such was the case with Jim Fixx. His autopsy, conducted by the chief medical examiner of Vermont, Dr. Eleanor McQuillen, showed that his coronary arteries were severely obstructed by arteriosclerosis, or clogging through the build-up of fatty substances. Specifically, there was extensive blockage of three vessels in Jim Fixx's two coronary arteries, those crucial channels supplying blood to the physical structure of the heart. In medical terms, the clogging occurred in the left circumflex and left anterior descending coronary arteries, and also in the right coronary artery (see Figure 1).

The branches of these slim, short arteries loop and wind around the front part of the heart. They act as a lifeline conveying freshly pumped blood from the heart right back into the heart tissues. The coronary vessels are crucial to maintaining life. If even one of them becomes blocked by fatty deposits so that it can't transport blood to the heart muscle, the tissues that this artery serves may die.

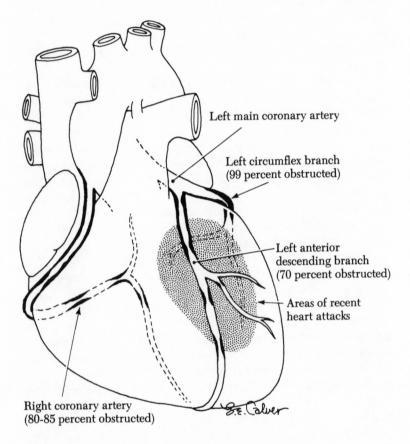

Left main coronary artery

Left circumflex branch
(99 percent obstructed)

Left anterior
descending branch
(70 percent obstructed)

Areas of recent
heart attacks

Right coronary artery
(80-85 percent obstructed)

Figure 1. Blood Supply to Jim Fixx's Heart at His Death

That's what a heart attack is all about—the death of heart tissue. If the death of heart cells is too extensive, the entire heart pump may cease to function. Sudden death will be the result.

In Jim Fixx, one section of the left coronary artery, the left circumflex, was almost completely blocked off by fatty deposits. In fact, there was only a "pinpoint" opening remaining. Another branch, the left anterior descending artery, was about 70 percent narrowed by the "hardening" or clogging process. The right coronary artery was also severely clogged, with 80 to 85 percent obstruction.

This "hardening" or clogging of the coronary arteries with cholesterol "garbage," or plaque, is always a time bomb. It was almost certain that there would be a lethal explosion in Jim's system unless steps were taken through surgery or a change of lifestyle to reduce the risk that he faced. Those steps were never taken.

After this arteriosclerosis had progressed to highly dangerous levels, other even more ominous events began to occur. Jim suffered at least three mild heart attacks prior to the cardiac event that killed him on Route 15 in Vermont. His autopsy revealed scar tissue on three parts of his heart tissue—a sure indication that other myocardial infarctions, or heart attacks, had occurred before the one that killed him. One of the attacks occurred about two weeks before his death; another occurred about four weeks before he died. Still another probably struck no earlier than about eight weeks before that fatal run in Vermont.

Was there any signal that he was having those prior heart attacks when they hit?

That's a difficult, if not impossible, question to answer because of the slight evidence we have. But let me give it a try. Jim was on vacation on Cape Cod with family members during the month immediately preceding his death, and at that time, he was about as active as ever. He ran four races, including one of 12 miles and one of 5 miles, in those last few weeks. Also, just the day before he set off on his final trip to Vermont, he beat his younger sister Kitty handily at singles in tennis.

Yet even during this vigorous period, there were some signs that all might not be well. During the last month of his life, Jim mentioned to several people that he had experienced a tightness in his chest. It was variously described as a "tightness" at the base of the throat when he wasn't exercising, or a tightness at his sternum (breastbone) when he was four or five minutes into a run.

While I was discussing this subject with Jim's 23-year-old son, John, he recalled a run that he and his dad made during the month that the family was at the Cape. They were planning to run 8 miles, but after only about ten to fifteen minutes into the run, Jim told John that he had to stop and go to the restroom.

There was a small airport nearby, and they decided to walk over there so that Jim could use those facilities. But on the way, the two ran into the airport manager and began chatting with him. About ten minutes later, Jim told his son that he was ready to go again. But after a few seconds into the run, John asked, "Dad, I thought you had to go to the restroom?"

Jim responded, "No, I really didn't need to."

In medicine, we call this "window shopping angina." A patient with heart disease will experience chest pain while walking but won't want his companions to know he's having a problem. So he will stop momentarily to "window shop" until the chest pain disappears. Then, walking can be resumed without discomfort.

It seems to me that this is additional evidence that Jim Fixx was having more severe chest discomfort than he would admit to his family. But he was concerned enough about the sensations in his chest that he got on the phone while his family was with him at the Cape and asked a physician friend about the problem. They talked for a few minutes, and when Jim hung up, he said, "It's not something to worry about."

But it may have been something to worry about.

Any pain or tightness in the chest area during endurance exercise could have been angina pectoris—pain caused by a spasm of one of the coronary arteries of the heart. Furthermore, any discomfort that had occurred in his lower throat or chest when he wasn't exercising might even have been a mild heart attack. After all, we know from the autopsy that he had suffered at least three heart attacks about two, four, and eight-plus weeks prior to his death. So at least two must have occurred while he was vacationing on the Cape.

Jim thus may have had some slight signs of coronary artery trouble. But there was absolutely no indication of still another major threat that he faced. You see, in addition to his arteriosclerosis and the prior mild heart attacks, he also had an abnormally enlarged heart—much larger than might be expected in a well-conditioned distance runner.

What made Jim's heart so big? Simply this: He had a condition, probably one he was born with, involving "hypertrophy," or an enlargement of the septum and the four chambers in the heart. An abnormal thickening of the septum has often been associated with sudden death in athletes less than thirty years of age. In fact, as we'll see shortly, it might even be considered a leading candidate for the cause of Jim's death.

These, then, are the three crucial internal physiological factors that most likely contributed to Jim Fixx's death: advanced arteriosclerosis; a series of recent prior heart attacks; and a congenitally enlarged, diseased heart. Truly a terrible triumvirate.

But even with these problems, was Jim's death inevitable? Despite the sad state of his heart and arteries, was there anything he might have done to postpone that final date with death?

Obviously, there were limits to what he could do to overcome his genetic predisposition to heart trouble. His enlarged heart was a "given," a condition Jim may have inherited. Also, his clogged arteries and the series of recent, mild heart attacks may be traced in part to an inheritance over which he had no control.

To put it bluntly, Jim Fixx had an exceptionally ominous family history that made him a leading candidate for death at an early age. On November 19, 1942, Jim's father Calvin Fixx, a member of the editorial staff of *Time*, suffered a massive heart attack in New York City. He was immediately rushed to Lenox Hill Hospital, where he was placed in an oxygen tent and kept under medical supervision for a number of weeks.

Calvin was only thirty-six years old.

After he returned home, he had to be quiet for a month, and he didn't go back to work for about a year. The family moved down to Sarasota, Florida, where they hoped Calvin would recuperate more quickly. He did seem to do well in a warmer climate. But before long, he returned to the stressful New York publishing scene, and the stage was soon set for tragedy.

Almost exactly seven years after his first heart attack, Calvin's health began to go downhill again. But he kept working hard in the high-pressure world of New York publishing. One day, he wrote a speech for a corporate executive and then attended the event in Atlantic City, New Jersey, where the speech was to be given. While he was still in New Jersey, his wife, Marlys, got a call from him.

"Would you like to come down here?" he asked.

Sensing something was wrong, she went to him immediately. Sure enough, when she first saw him at the hotel, she knew he should be in a hospital. Without delay, she had him placed under medical care, but he passed away shortly afterward of another heart attack.

At his death, Calvin Fixx was only forty-three years old.

Jim Fixx, who admired his father greatly, was always conscious that the older man had died of heart disease at a very young age. In fact, when Jim became forty-three in 1975, he noted that this was "the age my father had been when he died."

With an almost audible sigh of relief, Jim observed, "Thereafter, it no longer struck me as unseemly or disrespectful to try to do more than he had done. Soon, after all, I would be older than he was— older than my own father! I felt a new freedom to work more purposefully than I previously had" (*Jackpot!*).

It may have been more than coincidence that Jim Fixx began running seriously when he was approximately thirty-six, or about the age when his father had suffered his first heart attack.

On the brighter side, Jim could be encouraged by the fact that there was also a lot of longevity in his family. His mother is still alive, and his paternal and maternal grandparents lived to ripe old ages, some well up into their nineties.

But still, there was the fact of his father's death. This was a haunting presence that simply couldn't be glossed over, either by the heritage of other relatives or by Jim's increasingly healthy lifestyle. He correctly recognized that even one tragic event in his family history could have deadly consequences for his own health.

There's no question that the genetic predisposition to develop heart disease can be passed from father to son. In fact, if an autopsy had been done on Calvin Fixx, it's likely the coroner would have discovered a pattern of arteriosclerosis similar to that which was found more than three decades later in his son. I find myself wondering if the autopsy would have revealed a congenitally enlarged heart, like the one Jim had. That's a provocative question which, to my knowledge, cannot be answered.

Family history, then, was perhaps the key factor in Jim's background, propelling him toward his premature death. At the same time, there are other factors that can hasten or retard the inexorable, fateful march of heredity. Unfortunately, in Jim's case the negative factors far outweighed the positives.

For one thing, Jim had been under considerable stress for years prior to his death, and he didn't handle the stress well. Before he became one of the most successful authors of all time, Jim Fixx rose to the top of the magazine editing field. In 1967, he was promoted to managing editor of *McCall's,* which then had the third largest circulation of any American magazine. He later worked as a writer for *Life* and held other high-level editorial posts.

But according to his family, Jim wasn't very happy. He had been through a divorce, which is always listed by medical experts as one of life's most stressful events. He had also switched jobs several times, an experience that tends to cause great stress. Finally, he generally felt unfulfilled.

"For nearly ten years . . . I was bored and restless," he wrote of his life from the mid-sixties to the mid-seventies. "The work I was doing wasn't what I wanted to do, and I therefore did not do it very well. . . . I had a mortgaged house, four children and a wife, not to mention a former wife, for whom I was required to provide some $12,000 a year" (*Jackpot!*).

After he was fired from his last editing job, he decided to concentrate on freelance writing. Soon, he had a contract to write a book on his favorite avocation, running. The result was *The Complete Book of Running*.

There was tremendous satisfaction for Jim in the writing and financial success of this great bestseller. But success was a two-edged sword. Achievement brought greater fulfillment and independence; at the same time, it ushered in increasing pressures.

To meet the expectations of his publisher and his public, he had to promote the book in major national radio, television, and newspaper interviews. Regrettably, however, Jim didn't thrive in the public eye. He got increasingly nervous and uncomfortable when interviewed.

Finally, he suffered some sort of major anxiety attack before a scheduled appearance on the "A.M. Chicago" talk show in November 1977. His heart began to pound wildly, he got dizzy, and finally he asked the interviewer to terminate the interview because he didn't feel well enough to continue.

Nor were his pressures limited to public appearances. Shortly after he was featured in *People* magazine, thieves broke into his home and stole jewelry, silverware, and other valuables. Not an easy experience for anyone. And especially not so easy for a fundamentally private person, who would have preferred to be off by himself or with a small group of family and friends.

To counteract the anxiety he was feeling, Jim wrote in *Jackpot!* that he began to take Valium before his speeches and other public appearances. That may have helped him somewhat. But still, the other pressures mounted: a second divorce; a loss of $50,000 in investments he had made with his new wealth.

He kept a regular journal of his thoughts and feelings, and in that record there are indications that his anxieties continued in one form or another, right up to that final vacation on Cape Cod. His mother, who has read the latest journal entries, said, "There is a mention of anxiety before he spoke on television, and before he spoke to audiences of up to a thousand people. He never quite got over that feeling of real anxiety. He said his heart would race, and he felt extremely tense. And nervous."

Jim would say to his loved ones, "I just don't want any more of these talks. I don't want any more of these appearances."

But then, because he was in such demand, something would always come up. A persuasive promoter might offer a fascinating new deal, or a journalist would contact him for an interview. And he would be back at it again, on the air or otherwise before the public.

Stress over a period of years—especially stress that a person is not handling well—is a major factor associated with heart disease. It seems clear that Jim had far too much stress and fatigue in his life, right up to the moment that he set out on that final run in northern Vermont.

But excessive stress wasn't the only problem with the way he led his life. He also had been a heavy smoker for years before he started running. Until the 1964 Surgeon General's report on smoking and health, Jim was smoking two packs of cigarettes a day.

As he got more serious about running, he dropped smoking. But this habit may very well have helped lay down the basis for his advanced case of arteriosclerosis. An overwhelming number of scientific studies show that smoking cigarettes greatly increases a person's chances of getting heart disease.

Researchers from the Medical College of Wisconsin reported in the November 8, 1984, issue of the *New England Journal of Medicine* that heavy smoking may cause cardiomyopathy, a condition in which the heart enlarges because of decreased ability of the muscle to contract. It's been known for years that smoking can cause heart attacks indirectly by interfering with blood supply. But the Wisconsin team contends that the chemicals in smoke cause diffuse damage throughout the heart.

Their conclusion: "Smoking increases the risk of heart attacks in part by causing deposits which occlude the arteries in the heart. But there also appears to be a second mechanism. Smoking may change certain components of the blood, making it more likely for a blood clot to form in the arteries."

Smoking also tends to enhance cholesterol deposits in the coronary arteries, perhaps by reducing the level of "good" cholesterol (high density lipoprotein, or HDL) in the blood. The HDL cholesterol probably acts as a kind of garbage removal device to get rid of dangerous fatty substances in the blood. If you don't have enough HDL cholesterol, you're more likely to develop hardening of the arteries. This may be the reason that smokers are known to be more susceptible to developing arteriosclerosis than nonsmokers.

Another deficiency in Jim's prerunning lifestyle was that he had been quite sedentary. Furthermore, too much good food and drink had caused his body to balloon, so that he was about sixty pounds overweight. Jim had always played some tennis, a sport he had enjoyed since his days on the team at the Trinity School, a prep school in New York City. But tennis is not the most efficient sport for developing cardiovascular fitness and holding down a person's weight.

Jim himself confessed in one of his writings that he soared up from a weight of 170 in his teens to nearly 214 in 1968, when he was thirty-six years old. In some interviews, he said he got as high as 220. The weight gain had been gradual, and Jim attributed it to his sedentary lifestyle as an editor. He had simply indulged in too many extravagant, martini-laden lunches.

After he started running, his weight gradually declined to about 160 or 165, though it could creep up to about 170. He wrote in *Jackpot!* that he turned in his worst performance in five years in the 1977 New York City Marathon. He blamed the "sedentary labor of writing a running book" for his lessened cardiovascular fitness. Also, he wrote, "The doughnut of flab that has congealed around my midsection is, I suspect, partly responsible."

Jim's autopsy showed that he weighed approximately 170 pounds at his death—or somewhat heavier than he would have liked.

Obesity is a major factor associated with heart disease and a shortened life span. So Jim's extremely overweight condition, which developed during the decade or two before he began running and eating better, may also have helped lay the groundwork for the heart disease that finally killed him.

Clearly, Jim's way of living before he embarked on a running regimen meant he had several strikes against him: Excessive stress, heavy smoking, sedentary living, and obesity—when combined with his heredity—*had* to encourage coronary artery disease. But there was still another factor, one well within his control, which may literally have made the difference between life and death. This was the fact that he never underwent regular, comprehensive medical examinations and never had a *maximal* stress test.

All of the reports released following Jim Fixx's death indicated that he never had either a complete medical exam or a stress test. Also, in his books, the most recent medical exam of any type he mentioned was one he had in the late 1960s following a tennis injury. But in fact, his son Paul found, in perusing his personal records, copies of a physical exam with a submaximal stress test dated June 12, 1973. Furthermore, there were indications of heart abnormalities (from the resting ECG) which may have been associated with his death. Yet, for some reason, he failed to act on these findings with follow-up exams.

Specifically, Jim went in for a treadmill stress test in 1973 because he was writing an article on the subject—at least that's what the medical records indicate. During the test, he exercised to a heart rate of 167, which was considerably below his predicted maximum heart rate of 185. (He was forty-one years old at the time.)

The report on the test said that the results were "negative"—that is, there was no sign of any cardiovascular problem. Also, the report stated that his level of fitness was "high." By our standards at the Aerobics Center, he would have been in the "good" category of fitness. This result could well have been misleading, however, because the test was performed only to a submaximal level. Consequently, it may have missed heart abnormalities that might have appeared if the test had been maximal. Also, the state of the stress-testing art in 1973 was such that the equipment and procedures might have been unable to pick up some problems.

Even more significant than the stress test results were the results of the physical exam and resting ECG that Jim had before taking the test. A chest X-ray indicated he might have an enlarged heart. Listening to the heart with a stethoscope revealed two heart murmurs, one in the center of the chest and the other on the lower left side. Both of these murmurs, though they were designated "functional" or benign, are at times found with an enlarged, diseased heart. And the resting electrocardiogram was abnormal, showing a "right axis deviation" and possible right ventricular hypertrophy—again, an indication of an enlarged heart. One of our cardiologists at the Aerobics Center, Dr. Jim Farr, in evaluating Jim Fixx's resting ECG, confirmed that the tracings could be consistent with several abnormalities: right axis deviation ($+150°$); right ventricular hypertrophy; antecedent true posterior myocardial infarction; and other peculiarities associated with heart enlargement.

Treadmill stress testing was in its infancy when Jim was tested back in 1973, and the field of cardiology has also developed considerably since that time. But even with these limitations and even though his stress test report came back negative, he was advised to have a follow-up exam with his physician to check out the other abnormalities. And he failed to do it.

There's a great likelihood that if Jim had gone back for further testing in 1973, his problems might have been picked up. Moreover, if in later years he had gone in for regular, complete physicals with maximal stress testing, there's no question in my mind that his heart abnormalities would have been detected—and probably his life saved.

I have made this point many times since Jim's death, and both professional and lay people have asked me, "How can you be so sure that the test would have been abnormal?" Unfortunately, I can't say for sure that it would have been abnormal. But I have seen many patients with terribly abnormal stress electrocardiograms whose coronary arteriograms revealed much less disease than Jim Fixx had.

To illustrate this point in very personal terms, I want to share with you an experience I had with Robert E. Hood, a 58-year-old friend whose life and condition closely parallel that of Jim Fixx. Hood, the editor of *Boys' Life* magazine, was preparing an article on the Aerobics Center for publication in his magazine. During his research, he was given a treadmill stress electrocardiogram—his first ever!

The test results were clearly abnormal. Since he was not having any symptoms of heart disease, however, he was enrolled in our supervised cardiac rehabilitation exercise program. Shortly afterward, he took a second treadmill stress test. The abnormality which showed up on the first test had not improved, and so he was encouraged to

have a coronary arteriogram, or heart catheterization. By this procedure, dye was injected into his coronary arteries so that an X-ray
could be made to show their condition.

The result? The arteriogram showed Bob had coronary artery
disease even more severe and extensive than that found in Jim Fixx.
There were five places where the blockages ranged from 80 to 95
percent! Bob could have undergone a surgical bypass procedure. But
because he had little angina, and because he could be closely supervised in our cardiac rehabilitation program, he was allowed to pursue
a nonsurgical approach. This included drugs, a low-cholesterol diet,
and regular, *moderate* aerobic exercise.

Specifically, Bob was given drugs to control his pulse rate and
blood pressure and to dilate the arteries. Also, he received a medication designed to stop further clogging in his arteries. The diet we put
him on prohibited eggs, dairy products, fried foods, and most red
meat. As for exercise, he worked up to running three miles in thirty
minutes, five days a week.

Of course, there were some things about Bob Hood that distinguished him from Jim Fixx. For one thing, Bob has never smoked.
Also, he says he's had no particular problems with obesity or stress.
But Bob Hood's heredity presents a more disturbing picture: Several
of his close relatives have a history of heart disease and have suffered
early heart attacks.

The key point in any comparison is this: Bob Hood had at least as
serious a case of arteriosclerosis as Jim Fixx. Also, he had some of the
same risk factors as Fixx, with no particular symptoms that gave him
any warning there was a problem.

Furthermore, like Fixx, Bob would probably have continued living and behaving as he had always done—*except for the fact that he
took a stress test* and acted on the results. That test showed that he
would be heading for big trouble unless he took some decisive steps
to save himself. He chose the nonsurgical route that was available.
Now, some five years later, he's alive and vigorously active. (Remember, too, that running 15 ten-minute miles per week is much less of a
strain on a diseased heart than running seventy, seven- to eight-minute miles a week, as Jim Fixx did.)

These, then, are some of the negative health factors that probably contributed to Jim's heart disease. As we recount them in all

their deadly detail, it may seem overwhelmingly obvious that the major source of his problem was progressive hardening of the arteries. But still, there are some facts about Jim Fixx that don't fit quite so neatly into the coronary disease equation.

Take his cholesterol, for example. Jim had a high level of cholesterol in his blood—slightly more than 250 according to two separate measurements toward the end of his life. At the same time, however, he had an extremely *healthy* ratio of total cholesterol to "good" (high density lipoprotein) cholesterol—at least during the last few years of his life. (See Chapter 4 for a more extensive discussion of this topic.)

Jim was well aware of the importance of a person's cholesterol readings in predicting arteriosclerosis. Specifically, he kept close watch over his total cholesterol and had it checked on a number of occasions. Even more important, he understood the importance of the ratio of total cholesterol to "good" cholesterol. For men, this ratio should be less than 5.0 and preferably less than 4.5. Women should keep the ratio at least at 4.5, and preferably 4.0. If it's higher, the chances increase that hardening of the arteries is occurring.

Jim told several family members that he had gone to have his cholesterol checked and that it was "okay." Specifically, he wrote Peggy (Lillis) Palmer in 1980 that his total cholesterol was 253 and his HDL cholesterol was 87. This would have given him a total cholesterol/HDL cholesterol ratio of 2.91—truly an excellent reading. The autopsy revealed that Jim's total cholesterol just after death was 254, and his HDL cholesterol was 73. Once again, the ratio of 3.48 was quite good.

In addition, Jim's triglyceride readings, another indication of fatty substances in the blood, were at a rather low, and therefore healthy, level. He came in with a value of 57 in 1980, and his autopsy showed that they were 109 at the time of his death. At our clinic, triglycerides of 115 or below don't even qualify as a risk factor for heart disease. So Jim was in good shape in this area, as well as with his cholesterol—though admittedly, I do encourage my patients to work toward a cholesterol level of less than 200 and triglycerides less than 100.

What should we conclude from the total picture presented by these laboratory findings?

Several things pop into my mind. First of all, even though Jim's blood-fat readings were acceptable later in life, I wonder what they were like in those years before he started running? By the accounts of those close to him, Jim ate "very high-fat foods" before he got into running in his late thirties. He was a steak-and-potatoes man, and he also liked shrimp, lobster, and other rich foods. Probably, his cholesterol count was much higher in those days, and probably he was developing severely clogged arteries.

After Jim became deeply committed to running, his diet changed. He ate little for breakfast and lunch. Maybe a piece of toast smeared with peanut butter and some fresh grapefruit in the morning. Then, some yogurt or sardines for the noon meal.

He would have his evening meal at about 7:00 P.M., after he had gone for his run, and then he would really load up on food: He preferred salads and dishes high in complex carbohydrates, like fruit, vegetables, and pasta. Grilled fish was another favorite. Also, anchovies in olive oil. Typically, he would wash it all down with a few glasses of wine. Frequently, when he was visiting his mother, he would get so sleepy after that heavy evening meal that he would head for bed about 8:30 P.M.

From what I can tell, Jim was on a reasonably good diet in the final years of his life, though a strict, no-fat diet would probably have been best of all. Also, at the Aerobics Center, we recommend that a person's calories be weighted more toward the morning and noon meals, both for better nutritional balance and to control weight more effectively.

Let me sum up this cholesterol discussion simply by saying you can't rely on one risk factor or one limited set of steps to determine whether or not you have heart disease. By looking only at his cholesterol readings, you might think it would be unlikely for Jim to have a problem with clogged arteries. But when you look at other factors, such as family history, high stress levels, years of smoking, and prior obesity and sedentary living, you can't be quite so sure. The best way for anyone to understand exactly what impact all these factors have had or are having on the internal circulatory system is to have a complete physical examination, including blood studies and treadmill stress testing.

These, then, are some of the main facts about Jim Fixx and his health. What exactly do they tell us about the probable cause of his death? Three viable possibilities emerge from the evidence we have available:

- Jim died from a cardiac irregularity, secondary to one or more recent heart attacks caused by an inability of the blood to get to the heart through multiple clogged coronary arteries.
- Jim died from a sudden cardiac irregularity caused by the decompensation of an abnormally enlarged, diseased heart—a condition he may have had since birth.
- Jim died from a fatal shortage of blood to the heart, which occurred after he fainted from an inadequate, post-exercise cooldown.

Now, let's examine each of these possible explanations in greater detail.

The Clogged Artery Cause

This explanation of Jim Fixx's death is the one accepted in the Vermont autopsy report. The chief medical examiner says that the death event began with a "sudden cardiac arrhythmia while jogging." This means that his heart started beating irregularly at some point during the last part of his run.

The irregularity, the chief medical examiner writes, resulted from "severe coronary arteriosclerosis with myocardial infarction of the posterior and postero-lateral left ventricle." In lay terms, this means that the irregularity of heartbeat was caused by a failure of the blood to get to the heart muscle through the clogged coronary arteries. As a result of the lack of blood, the left ventricle or lower chamber of the heart was so severely damaged that death resulted.

The sequence of events might have gone like this: As we know, Jim was quite tired when he started out on his run. He probably wanted to run his usual ten miles before dinner. But by jogging up and down those Vermont hills, he got himself into an excessively fatigued state. Realizing that he would never make his daily mileage goal, he turned back after going about two miles out on Route 15.

But the tiredness increased and when he was within a couple of hundred yards of the motel, an excessively high heart rate, called "ventricular tachycardia," set in. His heart was racing at somewhere between 250 and 300 beats per minute, or well above the 150–160 rate that would probably have been normal for his runs. Also, there may have been some irregularity to his heart rhythm. (See Figure 2.)

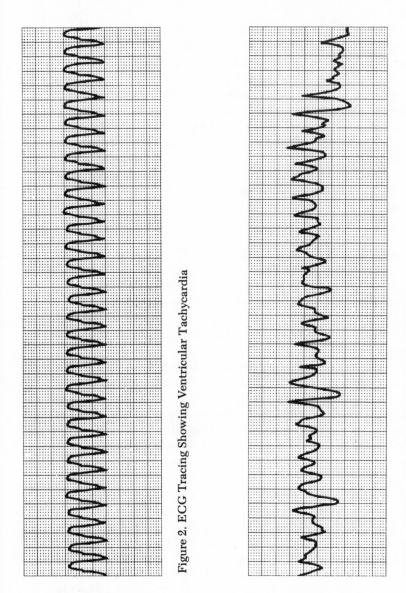

Figure 2. ECG Tracing Showing Ventricular Tachycardia

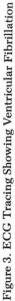

Figure 3. ECG Tracing Showing Ventricular Fibrillation

By now, Jim must have known something was seriously wrong. His goal would probably have been to get back to the motel as quickly as possible and allow his body to return to normal. But that wasn't to be. The heartbeat grew wilder and wilder.

Jim soon became nauseous and light-headed because of the fast, irregular heartbeat. The heart was now operating quite inefficiently. It wasn't pumping very well, and this meant that too little blood and oxygen were being transported to the heart tissues. At this point, the clogged coronary arteries—ravaged by the potentially deadly arterio-sclerosis—began to make things much worse. They prevented more blood from getting to the lower left side of his heart.

Also, there was still another lethal factor at work. As you'll re-member, Jim had suffered three prior heart attacks, two of them within two to four weeks of this incident on the Vermont road. Con-sequently, his heart would have been less efficient and more irritable because the damaged tissues from those other attacks would not have healed completely.

In fact, those recent heart attacks could have been the cause of the fatal heartbeat irregularity. That's why hospitals monitor heart attack victims in coronary care units. They want to be able to shock or defibrillate them immediately if the newly damaged heart goes into a dangerous, irregular beat. Yet these irregularities in the heartbeat most often occur during the first forty-eight hours after a heart attack.

So Jim's heart was in critical need of blood and oxygen; in medi-cal terms, it had become what we call "ischemic." But relief was out of reach. As he reached the steep, grassy hill just across from the Village Motel, the fast, irregular heartbeats went completely out of control.

He probably stopped in the hope that the symptoms would pass. But it was too late. He collapsed to his knees and slumped over against the embankment next to the road. This was about the time that his heart began to flutter irregularly in what's called "ventricular fibrillation." (See Figure 3.) The victim slips into unconsciousness immediately in such cases, and death occurs within three to five min-utes unless resuscitation can be started.

As a precedent for this sequence of events, let me take you back to a race I was monitoring in 1975. It was a two-mile event for men over forty and was being run in progressively faster heats. Approxi-mately 200 yards from the finish of one of the slower heats, I noticed that an older gentleman, who was sixty-one years old at the time, was apparently having some difficulty running. He didn't fall and was able to complete the run, but then he collapsed, unconscious, at my feet.

A rapid evaluation I made revealed no pulse; then the man began to go into convulsions. Immediately, I placed the monitoring electrocardiographic paddles on his chest, and I could see that he was already in ventricular fibrillation, that potentially fatal, fluttering heartbeat. But we had reached him in time. Two electrical shocks from a defibrillator we had on hand brought him back to consciousness.

He was then taken on to the hospital for observation, and twenty-four hours later, he was discharged without ever showing any signs of a new or old heart attack. The man had no residual effects from this incident, but about two years later, he did have coronary artery bypass surgery for underlying arteriosclerosis.

Interestingly, when I discussed this experience with the man, he couldn't recall any part of the last 200 yards of that race! I'm convinced that he was in ventricular tachycardia for at least a part of that time, and this progressed into ventricular fibrillation and finally into unconsciousness by the end of the run.

As far as the Jim Fixx case is concerned, Vermont's chief medical examiner, Eleanor McQuillen, sums it up by saying, "Finally, running did not cause [his] death . . . severe and silent coronary arteriosclerosis did."

I agree with her that this was the most likely cause of death. Still, there are other possibilities that could have contributed to the demise of Jim Fixx, or may even have been the primary reason for his death.

The Enlarged Heart Explanation

The autopsy revealed that Jim had an extremely large heart—much larger than you would expect even in a highly conditioned marathon runner (see Figure 4). It weighed 575 grams, and by most estimates, a person of Jim's size and physical condition should have had a heart weighing no more than 400 to 450 grams (see Figure 5).

The reason for the enlargement, as we have seen, was a condition that he may have been born with, called "biventricular hypertrophy," or excessively large ventricles (lower heart chambers). Also, he had "asymmetric septal hypertrophy," or ASH as it's sometimes called. That means the wall separating the two lower chambers of the heart was unusually thick. (This condition is characterized by a ventricular septum thickness that is at least 1.30 times the thickness of the free left ventricular wall. Since the autopsy revealed a septal bulge that measured 2.8 centimeters and the remaining septum 2.2 centimeters, this gives a ratio of 1.87 or 1.47, since the free left ventricular wall was 1.5 centimeters thick [see Figure 4].)

His heart should be regarded as diseased because of this enlargement. As a result, it was more susceptible than the normal heart to serious health problems, including sudden death. (In retrospect, the resting ECG abnormalities, the enlarged heart noted on the chest X-ray, and the heart murmurs detected at the time of the physical examination in 1973 were all consistent with biventricular hypertrophy and ASH.) Studies of patients with this relatively rare heart disorder have revealed all sorts of abnormalities, such as electrical instability in the heart and the fatal fluttering movements (ventricular fibrillation) which can lead to death.

So in this particular scenario, Jim Fixx may have met his fate this way:

Problems with his enlarged heart could have struck him at any time in the years after he began long distance running. He was living under a death sentence. It just happened that the run he had chosen outside of Hardwick, Vermont, was to be his last. The other pressures that had been building up in him may have finally come to a head as he ran along Route 15. The stress was too much for his congenitally weak heart, with its unstable electrical activity and susceptibility to fatal fluttering.

As he was about to complete his run, with the Village Motel already in sight, he would have begun to feel chest discomfort, unusual shortness of breath, and a pounding heart. Then, he would have become light-headed, and to regain his equilibrium, he probably pulled up to a halt next to the steep grassy hill near the motel. Finally, Jim would have fainted. The final fluttering of his heart would have begun about this time. Sudden death would have occurred a few minutes later.

Some young athletes die of this condition or disease while they are playing sports. Tragically, the abnormality is difficult to detect and is usually diagnosed only at the time of an autopsy. But there are some medical procedures that may help a physician discover the abnormally enlarged heart.

For example, an electrocardiogram taken while the person is at

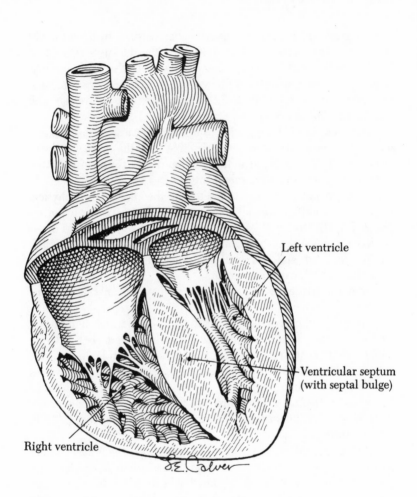

Left ventricle

Ventricular septum
(with septal bulge)

Right ventricle

Figure 4. Jim Fixx's Abnormal Heart, Showing Four Chamber
and Septal Enlargement

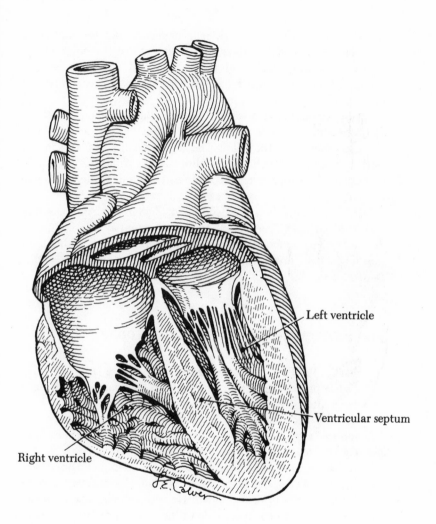

Figure 5. The Normal Athletic Heart

rest may be completely normal, *or* it may show some signs of heart enlargement, as it did in Jim's case. There is also the possibility of detecting the abnormality with the maximal performance stress electrocardiogram, during which test heart irritability or irregularity may be seen.

The best and easiest way to diagnose this condition is with an echocardiogram. This is an ultrasonic evaluation of the chambers, walls, and valves of the heart. The test is readily available in the cardiac section of most hospitals. Also, patients with this ASH condition usually have a particular type of heart murmur that can be identified at the time of a physical examination.

If an evaluation had revealed this problem in Jim Fixx, he would have been placed on medication to control potential heart irregularities and also on a much less strenuous exercise program. Either measure might have saved his life, if in fact the enlarged heart is what caused his death.

The Inadequate Cool-Down Catastrophe

Finally, Jim Fixx may have died simply because he failed to follow a basic procedure that he advocated in his books—an adequate cool-down after strenuous aerobic exercise.

The key fact in this possible scenario is that Jim Fixx came to a full stop just after he completed his run. Everything hinges on that. But what evidence do we have that he did stop?

According to witnesses questioned by Sgt. George F. Brierley of the Hardwick Police Department, Jim was initially discovered on his knees in a partially upright position. He was reclining against a very steep, grassy hill which rose up almost at right angles from the edge of the road where he had been running. His head was resting against the hill well above his legs, and his upper body lay at approximately a 45-degree angle to the road.

This position is important because it indicates, Sgt. Brierley believes, that Jim had stopped before he died. That conclusion also makes the most sense to me. If the heart attack had hit him while he was still running, his forward momentum would have caused his body to pitch forward, prone on the side of the road.

Also, some bystanders had started cardiopulmonary resuscitation procedures (CPR) on the road where they found Jim. Although these procedures were continued until he was pronounced dead at the hospital, both Sgt. Brierley and chief medical examiner McQuillen feel that Jim died shortly after he slumped to the ground.

Specifically, here is what might have happened: Jim completed his run just across the road from the Village Motel without any chest pains, light-headedness, or other symptoms. But for some reason, he came to a complete stop. He knew that proper cool-down procedures require walking or moving around briskly for three to five minutes after vigorous exercise. But still, he stopped.

Why did Jim stop? We can only speculate. Perhaps he stopped to wait for traffic before he crossed the road to the motel. Perhaps he pulled up to check his pulse rate, as many runners do. Or perhaps he just wanted to take a last look at the restful, bucolic scenery surrounding him before he went in for a shower.

The precise reason he stopped is not all that significant. But the *fact* that he stopped *is* important. By standing motionless, even for a few moments, Jim may have triggered a series of events that culminated in his death. As he came to a halt, about 60 percent of the blood in his body would have begun to "pool," or collect, below his waist. This customarily happens after a vigorous run. Simultaneously, the blood would have drained away from his heart and brain, and he would have become light-headed.

Then, his heart rate would have fallen rapidly—that's called "bradycardia," an abnormally slow heart rate. Jim would have quickly begun to get even more light-headed and nauseous, and before he was aware of what was happening, he would have lost consciousness. His blood pressure would also have fallen and triggered the production of adrenal hormones, which in such circumstances try to stimulate the heart to beat faster.

So now, Jim has crumpled down unconscious on the side of the road. But as fate would have it, he has fallen in the one spot on the road next to a steep hill. His head is resting well above his feet, and that fact alone may have triggered the events leading to his death.

You see, if he had fallen flat on the ground, with his head on a plane with or even below his feet, gravity would have allowed the blood to move naturally back to his heart. That's what happens with young soldiers who faint while they are standing at attention in a military formation. They pass out because the blood has settled in the lower part of their bodies. But then they usually snap right back after they have fallen flat on the ground. Unfortunately, circumstances conspired to keep Jim Fixx from that life-saving prone position.

The danger would have been aggravated by Jim's underlying arteriosclerosis. The cholesterol clogging in his vessels would have limited his ability to recover while in a semi-upright position on the ground. The blood just couldn't get back to his heart fast enough to sustain life. His blood pressure would still have been relatively low. His heart would have been beating rapidly but ineffectively. And all this time, gravity was adding to the problem, as the blood struggled unsuccessfully uphill toward his heart.

So Jim's heart and cardiovascular system, already weakened by prior heart attacks, by extensive arteriosclerosis, and perhaps by the congenitally enlarged condition, just couldn't compensate for that partially upright position into which he had fallen. His heart became starved for blood and oxygen.

Almost immediately, the heart either went into a cardiac arrest or the rate rose to a high, inefficient level, perhaps as fast as 250 beats per minute. The fatal fluttering, or ventricular fibrillation, followed. Now, little or no blood at all was getting to the heart. Within a short time, death would have occurred.

Although I lean toward the first explanation for Jim Fixx's death, either of the other two—or a combination of them—may have been the key cause. A recent South African study supports the possibility that a combination of coronary artery disease and an enlarged heart was the cause of Jim's death. (T.D. Noakes and A.G. Rose, "Exercise-related Deaths in Subjects with Coexistent Hypertrophic Cardiomyopathy and Coronary Artery Disease," *South African Medical Journal*, August 4, 1984.) The researchers documented three cases of exercise-related sudden deaths in white athletic men, aged twenty-eight, twenty-nine, and forty-two years, who had both problems (enlarged hearts and coronary heart disease). Two of the men were trained runners who had completed races of 90 kilometers (54 miles), and the third was a rugby player. Specifically, here's what happened to them:

- The 42-year-old man died suddenly in his sleep after running a 50-kilometer (30-mile) training run a few hours earlier.
- The 29-year-old died immediately after he had completed a 12-kilometer (7.2-mile) training run. He was resting on the ground

with his running partner when suddenly he lost consciousness and couldn't be revived.

- The 28-year-old was jogging with his wife in preparation for the next rugby season when he collapsed. He was dead by the time the doctor arrived.

Only one of these people, the 29-year-old, had any warning symptoms of ischemic heart disease.

In any event, in Jim Fixx's case there were several crucial factors in his background and his way of life that may have laid the groundwork for his death: the early death of his father; his obesity; unhealthy eating habits; heavy smoking; a stressful work environment; and his relatively sedentary existence until he was well into his thirties. These traits undoubtedly contributed to the poor state of his coronary arteries, as is the case with many young American men. Autopsies on American soldiers killed in Korea and in Vietnam revealed that 77 percent in Korea and 55 percent in Vietnam had some signs of coronary artery disease. In both cases, the average age of the soldiers examined was only twenty-two years.

By the time he started running at about age thirty-six, he may already have developed at least the severe level of clogging of his arteries that he had when he died, even though this was not detected at the time of his submaximal stress test in 1973. In fact, during the sixteen or so years that he was a serious runner, his arteriosclerosis may have stabilized or even have gotten better. Some studies of people who have quit smoking show that the clogging of their arteries with fatty deposits actually decreases.

But even with the dramatic change that occurred in his way of living and in his outward appearance, the way had already been paved for coronary danger and death. The only thing that perhaps could have stood between Jim and that final, fatal run would have been a clinical diagnosis of his condition. I believe that could definitely have been accomplished through a proper treadmill stress test and other medical evaluations. Unfortunately, with everything else he had done to improve his health, Jim failed to take this crucial step.

Whatever the complete answer to the question, "Why did Jim Fixx die?" there are many lessons to be learned from the death of this great runner and writer. Now, let's explore the first of those lessons— how *you* can reduce the risk of heart attack and sudden death, even as you get the maximum benefits from your aerobic exercise program.

CHAPTER THREE

WHY SUDDEN DEATH SOMETIMES STRIKES DURING AEROBIC EXERCISE

Sudden death is more common than you might think. It strikes 450,000 Americans each year, and that represents about 20 to 25 percent of all the annual deaths in the United States. Also, 40 percent of the victims of sudden death die of heart attacks.

When I talk about "sudden death," I am referring to death that occurs within six hours of the onset of symptoms. Although this definition accords with generally accepted standards established by the World Health Organization, there is some disagreement. For example, some researchers limit their understanding of sudden death to those fatalities that occur within one hour; others extend the limit as far as twenty-four hours. For present purposes, though, I'll stick with the six-hour definition.

But now, let's get more personal. What, you may wonder, is the relationship between abstract definitions and statistics about sudden death, and your own approach to exercise?

As we've already seen, the fact that you exercise doesn't automatically render you immune to sudden death. Certainly, there's no place in an intelligent health program for any Jim Fixx Syndrome, with a belief in "myths of invulnerability" for those who pursue regular aerobic activities. But even though exercise may not provide total protection, it doesn't necessarily place you more at risk, either. As a matter of fact, very few of the sudden deaths that take place each year occur during exercise. Furthermore, as we'll see later, an intelligent exercise program can help you avoid sudden death.

In the last decade, we've seen the interest in exercise reach a fever pitch. Hordes of enthusiasts have donned their sweatsuits or bathing trunks and headed for the nearest road, gym, or pool to work out. At the same time, however, a disturbing undercurrent of negativism and naysaying has emerged. Even as the ranks of exercisers grow, there are others who seem ready to implicate exercise as the prime culprit whenever sudden death strikes during these activities.

Reports of sudden death during exercise can be sensational—particularly when they involve a well-known sports figure like Jim Fixx or perhaps a popular teenager on a high school football team. Or take the case of the 48-year-old Frenchman, Jacques Bussereau, who died of a heart attack in the 1984 New York City Marathon. Headlines the next day screamed, "First Death Mars Race . . . One Runner Falls Dead . . . Frenchman Dies Of Cardiac Arrest . . . 1st Marathon Fatality."

The reports of these tragedies may often be quite accurate. But it's the interpretations that I get worried about, not the facts. Sports deaths can often be so misunderstood that they may call into question the basic benefits of aerobic exercise—an activity that has played a large role in the decline in deaths by heart disease during the past two decades.

As I see it, the potential risk to a small group who already suffer from heart disease is being so overstated that some healthy people feel a twinge of doubt as they stoop to put on their running shoes. While a few people may be wise to curtail vigorous exercise, the facts show that the great majority can continue to exercise without fear.

But what exactly are the facts? To answer this, let's explore some of the concrete evidence that has emerged in recent scientific studies.

Despite a flurry of reports about the potential dangers of exercising for some people, sudden death doesn't occur during sports nearly as often as you might think. In a review of international reports on sudden death, Jerry Goss in *Sportsmedicine* said that of 2606 sudden deaths examined in Finland, only twenty-two were associated with sports.

Those included sixteen with skiing, two with jogging, and four with other activities. To put this another way, among all the sudden deaths that occurred, sports were involved only 0.8 percent of the time. Not bad, when you consider that nearly three times as many sudden deaths, or 2.2 percent, occurred among Finnish sauna bathers!

Separate studies have confirmed these findings. In one, only eight sudden deaths occurred among 1,030,000 ski hikers in a sixteen-year period.

But when a person dies from a cardiovascular reason while running, it is immediately assumed that exercise caused the death. Yet if you look at the statistical probability of having a fatal heart attack by chance alone, the conclusions are most interesting. Koplan (*Journal of the American Medical Association*, Vol. 242, No. 23, December 7, 1979) concluded that if white male runners were nonsmokers at the lowest lean body weight who exercised for twenty minutes three times per week, then you would expect 4 deaths per year to occur from chance alone while they were running. If you add to the twenty minutes of running the two hours after running, another 30 deaths per year would be expected by chance alone. However, if runners were to resemble the standard white male population, you would expect 15 deaths to occur from cardiovascular disease each year while running and another 104 during the two hours after running. Consequently, 4 to 104 cardiovascular deaths per year are predicted on a purely temporal basis.

So, clearly, there is nothing inherently dangerous about exercise—as long as it's pursued intelligently. And being intelligent means having regular medical exams and then following your doctor's advice.

Also, there is some concern about strenuous exercise for *susceptible* people—that is, those with a high coronary risk profile, or those with existing coronary disease. These individuals naturally face a much higher risk of sudden death in any situation, whether they're exercising or not.

It's true, of course, that vigorous exercise may place undue extra stress on their hearts. But being susceptible to sudden death during exercise doesn't require you to be sedentary. Generally, people who have more risk factors, such as a family history of heart disease, excessive obesity, or a smoking habit, should first undergo a proper stress test. This way, they can see what sort of shape their hearts are in. Then, even if they have some sort of heart trouble, they may still be able to have an exercise program tailored to their personal needs by their physician.

Many who are interested in lowering their risk of sudden death first want to know whether there are any "low-risk" practices they can follow, and whether there are any "safe" sports they can play. They wonder, "When sudden death strikes during exercise, what exactly are the circumstances surrounding some of the tragedies? Also, what kinds of activities tend to be involved?"

Sudden death during sports usually happens within a few seconds. But as fast as these deaths may occur, they are typically the tragic culmination of long-term factors, which may have been at work for decades or even from birth.

For example, during one eighteen-month period, there were twenty-one sudden deaths reported among athletes in South Africa, and nineteen of those were probably cardiac-related. As we've learned from our discussion of the death of Jim Fixx, heart disease that eventually proves fatal may follow its deadly course for most of a person's life.

The sports in the South African study included rugby (seven deaths); refereeing (four); soccer and tennis (two each); golf, mountaineering, jogging, and yachting (one each). When researchers looked into the circumstances of these cardiac-related deaths, they found that the majority, like Jim Fixx, had advanced coronary arteriosclerosis or a personal history of heart disease. The remainder showed strong indications of heart disease through positive findings in exercise stress tests.

That's the bad news. The good news is that aerobic exercise such as swimming, cycling, and running can be helpful in modifying your overall risk of heart disease. This type of endurance exercise can help to counterbalance certain coronary risk factors that may contribute to coronary artery disease. Of course, aerobic exercise offers no absolute immunity against developing heart disease or experiencing sudden death. As we've already seen, even marathoners can develop arteriosclerosis and suffer sudden death when other risk factors are present.

So how can you use aerobic exercise safely to reduce your risk of sudden death?

First, it's important to find the proper intensity for your exercise routine. Of course, just how hard you should exercise is something only you and your doctor can determine. But remember: People at *all* levels of fitness may have a tendency to overdo it. Given his underlying coronary problems, Jim Fixx overdid it. A less strenuous program—say 15 instead of 60 to 70 miles a week—might have helped him avoid his fatal heart attack.

By the same token, people who are overweight, smoke heavily, or are generally sedentary during the week may be overdoing it when they exercise with racquetball or tennis just once a week. They should first alter their basic lifestyles; only then would they begin a regular exercise program, such as walking, thirty minutes a day four days a week. And they should only start after a thorough medical exam with a proper stress test.

So, when you consider the intensity at which you should exercise, it's important to consider your overall level of fitness and health. Even though some competitive runners may view with disdain their friends who jog along at a snail's pace, we must realize that vigorous exercise is not for everybody. In fact, *very* strenuous exercise—for more than a half hour a day, four or more days a week—is appropriate only for the very serious competitive athlete.

Even as I mention these caveats about the importance of exercise, however, I want to emphasize that intelligent exercise *must* be a key feature in any personal health program. Avoiding exercise completely can be as dangerous as doing too much. In short, it's better for your heart if you're active rather than sedentary. Exercise, particularly aerobic exercise, can help reduce overall risk of heart disease, because a sedentary lifestyle is a major coronary risk factor.

Exercise can also help counterbalance other factors that contribute to coronary disease. Of course, regular workouts can't completely eliminate all risk. We already know that from our discussion of the "myths of invulnerability" in the Jim Fixx Syndrome. In other words, exercise won't make a family history of heart disease disappear, nor will it wipe out an advanced case of hardening of the arteries.

But still, we can agree with Dr. Ben Hurley in the *Journal of the American Medical Association* that evidence is accumulating that aerobic exercise training "attenuates factors that promote atherosclerosis [arteriosclerosis]." That is, if you've got hardening of the arteries, a safe aerobic exercise program may help to slow, stop, or even reverse this condition.

Now, let's explore in a little more depth what it means to exercise safely. It comes as a startling revelation to some people that it's possible to exercise regularly without any discomfort and *still* be at risk. Nor is Jim Fixx the only illustration of this problem.

For example, in the South African study mentioned earlier, several referees were mentioned among the athletes who suddenly died. Most people don't usually realize how physically demanding refereeing can be, and that includes many of the referees themselves.

The reason I say that is because I've often seen overweight referees—particularly on the basketball court—sweating profusely as they run back and forth. Their tee shirts cling to their bodies, dripping wet, and their chests heave as they try to catch their breath. I often find myself wondering, "Just how wise is that?"

Without knowing anything else about some of these referees, I can see that they are already at risk simply by being overweight. And they would appear to be adding to the overall strain on their hearts with the stop-and-go activity of the game. I should hasten to say that some referees I know are trim and generally in better condition than most professional athletes.

Jim Tunney, the well-known National Football League referee, is a classic example of that statement. For five years he has been visiting our clinic on a semiannual basis. During that time, his treadmill performance has consistently ranked him in the top 2 percent of all 32,000 people tested at our clinic, regardless of age. To maintain that level of fitness, this 55-year-old man runs approximately three to four miles each day.

But the overweight, relatively inactive referees are another matter. They seem to be good examples of the possible consequences for people who exercise *despite* their poor overall level of fitness. After all, even a wisely constructed, regular program of exercise isn't necessarily going to erase a lifetime pattern of overeating and being out of shape.

Still, even though it's important to be prudent—especially if you're out of shape—it's also possible to overemphasize the occasional tragedies connected with a strenuous workout. Some critics of exercise have seized unfairly upon a few studies that appear to highlight the risk of sudden death among joggers and other exercisers.

In a six-year study of sudden deaths among joggers in Rhode Island, Dr. Paul D. Thompson found that the rate of death due to coronary heart disease among joggers was seven times that which could be expected from coronary heart disease among nonexercisers.

It's important to put such findings in perspective, however. For example, in this study, the total number of joggers who died suddenly in those six years was *only twelve!* And one of those victims died of an acute gastrointestinal hemorrhage, not from any heart problem. Finally, in the eleven other cases in the study, the primary cause of death was coronary heart disease—not something inherent in exercise itself.

I suppose it's possible to twist such studies into an indictment of exercise. But I don't see how an objective observer could come to such a conclusion. After all, it really shouldn't be too surprising that people with extremely advanced coronary heart disease may risk sudden death when they place excessive stress, such as vigorous exercise, on their already weakened hearts.

So, as some researchers have concluded, the death rate for persons who jog with advanced coronary heart disease may indeed be "seven times" the estimated death rate during less strenuous activities. But the number of such deaths is extremely small. And these findings only suggest that exercise contributes to sudden death in susceptible persons.

The main problem with any report about sudden death is that it usually commands a lot of attention and publicity. At the same time, it's easy for ill-informed critics to jump to a wrong conclusion, such as the notion that even moderate exercise may be bad for everybody.

But the hard evidence suggests that there's no need for the average exercise enthusiast to become alarmed. Even in the Rhode Island study just discussed, the researchers saw no great risk. With only one death per 7,620 joggers each year, the risk of exercise is actually quite small.

To emphasize just how small, the study said that the slight incidence of sudden death doesn't even justify such a small step as routine exercise testing of healthy people before they begin to train. I'm a little more cautious. To be on the safe side, I would always recommend that a sedentary person by age thirty-five, or at least by age forty, should have a treadmill stress test before beginning vigorous exercise.

So the risk of fatality during exercise in a person without symptoms is slight. But even so, the possibility still exists that some people will die. To understand better how this may happen and what you can do to reduce your own risks as much as possible, let's take a closer look at some of the main causes of sudden death in those who exercise.

Cause #1:   Hardening of the Arteries

Arteriosclerotic heart disease is the major cause of sudden death during exercise in adults. (In contrast, congenital cardiovascular disorders are the primary cause of death in younger patients.) But what sport is most likely to result in sudden death for those with this underlying coronary artery disease? The answer to this question isn't always so easy to predict. In another Rhode Island study of eighty-one people who died during recreational exercise, the largest number of deaths for any single activity, 23 percent, occurred during golf. Ironically, one of the least strenuous activities turned out to be the most "dangerous."

The next two activities were more strenuous. Jogging was second, with 20 percent; then came swimming, with 11 percent. But in an overwhelming 88 percent of all the cases, underlying arteriosclerosis, not exercise, was the primary cause of death. Most of these individuals, by the way, were people over age twenty-nine, and they had known heart abnormalities.

Tragically, most of the victims could have taken steps to save themselves if they had only been aware of what to do. According to the study, 93 percent of the arteriosclerosis victims had a medical history of heart disease or had some recognized risk factors. Their backgrounds strongly indicated that they were candidates for medical screening, which might have shown the presence of significant heart disease.

Yet those doing the study noted that only four of the people had undergone exercise testing! The researchers believe it's possible that if tests had been performed in many of the patients, the results might have indicated the need for more aggressive treatment prior to exercise.

So this second Rhode Island study concluded that death during recreational exercise is due mainly to arteriosclerosis. Also, the deaths tend to occur in individuals with recognized risk factors, known disease, and definite symptoms. Death during recreational exercise in patients without any symptoms is very unusual, the researchers said.

Finally, sudden death in people without symptoms or clear-cut coronary risk factors is relatively more frequent in younger age groups. With these younger people, the cause of death can often be traced to latent, congenital heart disorders.

What does all this have to say about you and your exercise program?

First of all, the researchers never say that exercise causes death. They do note, however, that exercise in persons with certain cardiac abnormalities can provoke an irregular heartbeat. This may increase the risk of sudden death. On the other hand, it's possible, according to the study, that these people would have died anyway, even if they had not exercised.

Secondly, certain types of exercise—namely, endurance activities like distance running, swimming, and cycling—are definitely more beneficial than others when it comes to modifying your overall risk. I suspect that further studies will confirm that people who participate primarily in less demanding weekend sports face higher risk of sudden death than those who run or swim regularly for moderate distances. Certainly, the previously mentioned Rhode Island study, where golfers were the group with the most sudden deaths, illustrates this point. Also, those who engage in certain kinds of nonaerobic exercise, particularly the type that requires occasional short, violent bursts of energy, such as weight-lifting, are probably at a much higher risk of dying suddenly with underlying arteriosclerosis.

In a report published in the October 4, 1984 issue of the *New England Journal of Medicine* ("The Incidence of Primary Cardiac Arrest During Vigorous Exercise"), the authors made it clear that the risk of primary cardiac arrest may be increased for a time during vigorous exercise. Yet among men with low levels of habitual activity, the relative risk of cardiac arrest during exercise was eleven times greater than it was among the men who were habitually active. In addition, among the habitually active, the overall risk of cardiac arrest was only 40 percent of that observed in the sedentary men.

Finally, remember that arteriosclerosis (or atherosclerosis—the words can be used interchangeably) may develop quite independently of your exercise program. Whatever your age, the disease is encouraged by risk factors such as smoking cigarettes, hypertension, high blood fats, diabetes, a family history of heart disease, or a high-stress lifestyle.

When you exercise in the presence of arteriosclerosis, your risk of

sudden death depends largely on the extent of the disease. To lessen
the risk of tragedy, researchers suggest that persons with high risk
factors for coronary artery disease should undergo treadmill stress
testing before starting their exercise program. Furthermore, persons
with known heart disease should exercise initially only under supervision in a coronary rehabilitation program. Their response will determine whether long-term supervision is necessary.

So far, we've seen that arteriosclerosis is the primary cause of
sudden death among exercisers. But it's not always to blame. In some
cases even where there were classic changes in electrocardiograms in
prior exercise testing, the athletes' coronary arteries were found to be
normal at the autopsy. Now, let's explore some of the other ways a
person may die without warning.

Cause #2:   Abnormality of the Internal Structure of the Heart

When a 37-year-old marathoner checked in at our clinic, he
seemed the picture of health. "No complaints from me, Doc," he
said. "I'm just here for my check-up."

On the face of it, he was the prototype of a person who runs ten
miles per day. His body was extremely lean, with only 8 to 10 percent
body fat. Blood tests were excellent, showing low levels of cholesterol.
He had a steady, low resting pulse, and he clocked an exceptional
thirty minutes on his Balke treadmill stress test.

Yet toward the end of the stress test, his heart rate leaped to
about 240 beats per minute. Sometimes, extremely high and irregular
heartbeats can occur in healthy people. At other times, however, they
are a signal of some dangerous underlying problem. We didn't want
to take any chances, so we ordered a few tests.

An echocardiogram, a special test that uses sound waves to provide a sonic picture of the heart, revealed that this runner did indeed
have a problem. He had a condition known by a medical mouthful—
"idiopathic hypertrophic subaortic stenosis," or IHSS; or in other
terminology, "hypertrophic cardiomyopathy," or HCM. To put it in
simple terms, there was a marked enlargement of an internal part of
his heart that caused an obstruction to blood leaving it. (See Figure
1.) In response to this obstruction, the heart adapted by enlarging the

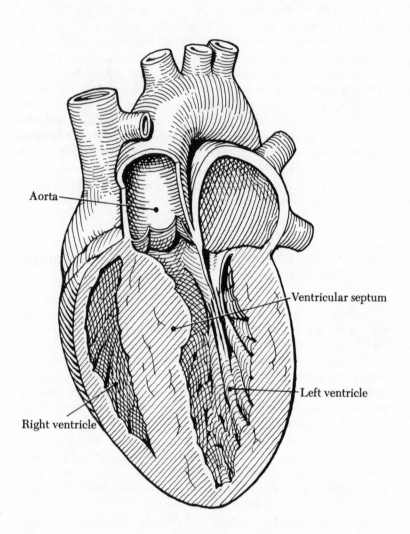

Figure 1. Idiopathic Hypertrophic Subaortic Stenosis (IHSS)

muscles of its main pump, the left ventricle. During peak demands such as during exercise, this obstruction prevented blood from getting out of the heart into the aorta and particularly into the coronary arteries. In serious cases, death can occur from this condition.

In general, symptoms associated with this condition include easy fatiguability, chest pain, some difficulty with breathing, near fainting or temporary loss of consciousness, heart palpitations, and an unusually fast or irregular heart rhythm. An electrocardiogram and/or a stress test may be of value in diagnosing this condition, as is listening to the heart. However, the echocardiogram (as it was in this case) is the most accurate test.

While exercise testing may be particularly useful in exposing a person's vulnerability to heart rhythm disorders, continuous ambulatory ECG monitoring can serve the same function. In one study, almost one-third of the patients with this condition had ECG abnormalities occur during the seventy-two continuous hours they were monitored. In addition, three-year follow-up studies revealed that those who showed ECG abnormalities during these tests had an increased risk of sudden death.

So, the situation this man faced was very serious. We had to tell him what can be the worst possible news to an avid runner: As a result of our diagnosis, we advised him to curtail or at least limit his exercise outings. Rather than run 50, 60, or even 70 miles a week as he was accustomed to do, we urged him to cut his weekly speed and distance to no more than a slow 12 to 14 miles. Finally, we told him to give up his stressful, competitive marathons. He was also given a medication to take four times a day.

He took the drugs, but that was as far as he was willing to go. He considered himself too much of a dedicated marathoner to swallow the entire preventive medicine "package" we had recommended. Because he was in the peak of health, he believed that his daily workout could only help to strengthen him. So, he ran another marathon later that year. According to family members, he wanted to "prove the doctors wrong."

The following spring, he returned to the clinic and took another treadmill stress test. Perhaps because of the medication he was receiving, he had a relatively normal ECG. Still, we repeated our advice to cut back on running. Even though his condition appeared to have stabilized, we knew that he was facing a serious risk.

But he continued to ignore all our advice. Later that spring, he participated in a triathlon—a three-phase race incorporating running, bicycling and swimming in a grueling test of endurance and fitness. It was then that more serious signals of his problem began to surface. During the bicycle phase, he tumbled off his vehicle and had to be revived by paramedics. The cause of the accident? A severe cardiac irregularity.

Although he was hospitalized for a short time, he rationalized his brush with death as being a result of heat stress and dehydration. Not only that, he steadfastly refused to accept the statement from the physician that he had experienced a high, irregular heartbeat—and that the condition could have killed him. Also, we told him once again to quit or at least cut back his running to a relatively few easy miles a week. But he still ignored our advice.

The next time he came to our clinic, he told us that he was continuing to run in marathons, and that the small irregularity in the stress tests really didn't bother him. Incredibly, he seemed to cling to the mistaken belief—one of those myths of invulnerability—that his running provided some kind of immunity from cardiovascular disease. He thought he could ignore these important symptoms.

As for his medication, he had found the four times a day regimen required on the previous prescription too hard to keep. To accommodate him, we changed his drug to one that he needed to take only once a day. Weeks later, we found out from his family that he had even decided to stop his new medication because, he said, it made him feel a little too "sluggish." Instead, he was going to try to continue his exercise program without any medication whatsoever.

One week after stopping his medication, he was training for yet another marathon by going on a seven-mile practice run. After running the course, he went into a restroom at a health club. Minutes later, one of the club employees noticed legs in an unnatural position beneath one of the stall doors. Quickly, the worker opened the door and found the 40-year-old marathoner—dead.

The autopsy revealed just what we suspected. His coronary arteries had no signs of arteriosclerosis whatsoever. But the autopsy did confirm that the IHSS was the cause of death. What's particularly tragic is that there were warning signs from the very first stress test. Had he followed our advice when his condition was first discovered, there is a good chance he would still be alive today.

It's often too late to wait for that "first sign of trouble." Many times, victims of sudden death get no warning whatsoever. They may believe that they will be well aware of the presence of heart disease through the classic symptoms of chest pain, shortness of breath, dizziness, and so on. But unfortunately, not everyone gets these symptoms. Even with classic hardening of the arteries, sudden death may be the first cardiac event in approximately 25 percent of the victims. With other heart problems as well, sudden death is frequently the first sign that something serious is wrong.

Cause #3:   An Abnormally Enlarged Heart, with Thickened Heart Tissue

This condition is one of the big physical problems Jim Fixx had, as we've already seen in Chapter 2. The other, of course, was hardening of the arteries.

The enlarged heart is characterized by ventricular enlargement and an unusual thickening of the ventricular septum, which separates the two lower heart chambers. This disorder, though rare, is the most common cause of sudden death among young, competitive athletes.

In the early 1960s, extensive large-scale studies of this problem were performed by the National Heart, Lung, and Blood Institute. Reports from this center indicated that almost one-half of the deaths in young athletes were from this enlarged heart disorder. In another study of sixty-two patients with this disorder, 40 percent of the deaths occurred during or just after vigorous activity. Fortunately, though, medications are available that reduce the risk associated with this problem. In thirty-six patients, aged fifteen to sixty-one years, who were followed for two to eight years, there were no deaths among twenty-two on medication. In contrast, there were four deaths among the fourteen control patients.

But as serious as this problem is, it can often be detected by certain tests—either a resting electrocardiogram or an echocardiogram. In a study of twenty-six persons who died suddenly, thirteen of the fatalities occurred during or immediately after physical exertion. The two key characteristics of this group were an abnormal electrocardiogram and a moderately to severely thickened ventricular septum.

As mentioned in Chapter 2, patients with this disorder may experience chest pain, unusually heavy breathing, a pounding heart beat, and even temporary loss of consciousness. Also, nearly all have a heart murmur that can be noted at the time of a physical examination. Some may be completely without signs or symptoms.

Under a doctor's care, tests such as ambulatory ECG monitoring, the echocardiogram, and the electrocardiogram can alert the physician to the presence of an enlarged heart. If the disease is relatively severe, the physician will recommend that the patient limit physical activity and be placed on medications that control heart irregularity. In some cases, a special type of surgery might be suggested if the response to medication is inadequate.

Finally, so you'll understand your physician if he's talking in technical terms, both Cause #2 (abnormality of the internal structure of the heart) and Cause #3 (the enlarged heart) are frequently referred to under the same name: "asymmetric septal hypertrophy" (ASH) or "hypertrophic cardiomyopathy" (HCM).

Cause #4:   Wrong Origin for Coronary Arteries

This problem arises when the left coronary artery begins at some point other than where it's supposed to begin on the aorta. (See Figure 2.) The frequency of sudden death from this condition is unknown, but in one study of young athletes, it accounted for 10.5 percent of the fatalities.

Here's how the problem develops: If the left coronary artery begins at a point where it gets pinched by the expansion of the aorta, strenuous exercise may cause a blockage and cut off the blood supply. Symptoms typically include chest pain and fainting.

This disorder may be detected through ECG abnormalities occurring during treadmill exercise testing or by taking a picture of the vascular system through a coronary arteriogram. If it's caught in time, the condition may be surgically corrected. But let me assure you, this condition is very rare.

Cause #5:   Inflammation of the Heart Muscle

Inflammation of the heart muscle, known technically as "myocarditis," may be caused by a viral infection such as influenza. Often,

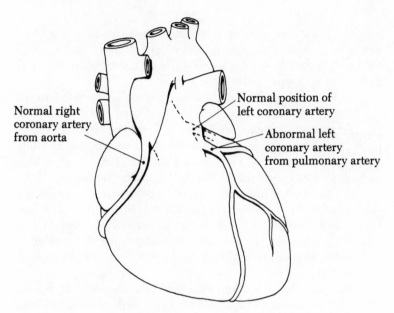

Normal right
coronary artery
from aorta

Normal position of
left coronary artery

Abnormal left
coronary artery
from pulmonary artery

Figure 2. Abnormal Origin of the Left Coronary Artery

the condition results in an irregular heartbeat, or "cardiac arrhythmia." Researchers believe that, in people with myocarditis, exercise can aggravate the irregularities of the heart. So exercising in an attempt to "sweat out" a fever-producing cold can be ill-advised.

Myocarditis can often be detected through changes in your electrocardiogram, though this test doesn't pick up the problem 100 percent of the time. Because of the potential for danger, I would advise you to avoid strenuous exertion during or immediately following a severe viral illness. Also, wait at least twenty-four hours after your temperature has returned to normal before resuming vigorous exercise.

Cause #6: Heart Valve Problems

Abnormal development of a heart valve can cause your doctor to hear odd sounds through his stethoscope—especially "murmurs" and "clicks." A heart murmur is a swishing sound caused as the blood moves in an unusual way through the various chambers and valves of the heart. A click is an extra sound the heart makes, often because a person has a "floppy" heart valve.

While rarely a cause of sudden death, abnormal heart valves can result in tragedy. One condition, called "prolapsed mitral valve," usually affects young women. (See Figure 3.) It may be characterized by chest pain, heart-pounding, or dizziness; or there may be no symptoms. The condition is also known by a number of other names, such as Barlow's Syndrome and the Mid-Systolic Click Syndrome.

This particular abnormality can often be detected by an electrocardiogram and usually does not prevent the patient from participating in sports. But if a person also has an accompanying symptom such as a racing heart—or what's called "supra-ventricular tachycardia"—a physician may recommend restricting activity, or prescribe medication, or both.

Even though there is the extremely rare possibility of sudden death in these cases, it's important not to get too worried if you have this condition. If you've been examined properly, the valve abnormality can be diagnosed through the echocardiogram. Furthermore, if a patient has no symptoms, it is not usually necessary to cut back on exercise. If symptoms do occur, they can usually be treated and you can keep on working out. The onset of symptoms is generally a sign that some modification in your activity may be necessary.

So these are a number of possible causes of sudden death which exercisers should understand. The common thread in following a safe program, whether you have one of these conditions or not, is to be stress-tested and otherwise thoroughly examined by a qualified physician. According to most researchers, treadmill exercise testing is one of the most helpful tests in determining the condition of your heart and coronary arteries.

Also, remember this: Even if you face some risk of coronary disease, you don't necessarily have to cut out exercise. You may just have to settle for an easier, more limited program than that pursued by people without any heart problems.

During a 65-month-long study of 2,935 adults at our Aerobics Center that was reported in the *Journal of the American Medical Association*, only two cardiac events occurred—and there were *no*

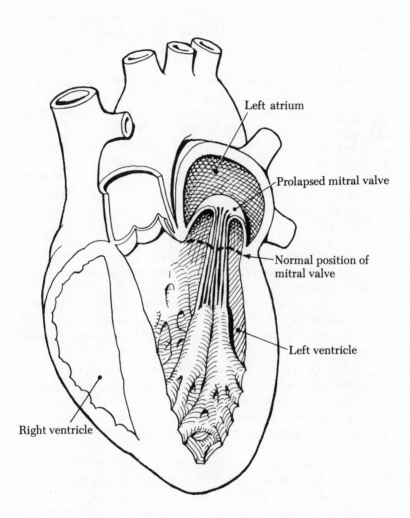

Left atrium

Prolapsed mitral valve

Normal position of
mitral valve

Left ventricle

Right ventricle

Figure 3. Prolapsed Mitral Valve

deaths. Since that time, the numbers have increased to more than 5,000 participants who have collectively run in excess of six million miles; and still, only the two nonfatal cardiac events have come to our attention.

Despite some popular reports that exercise risks may outweigh benefits, we found that no heart problems occurred in patients unless they were already suffering from some sort of heart disease. Often, that disease could be detected through routine tests.

We concluded that there was only a small risk of cardiovascular problems for adults participating in vigorous exercise *if* they had been screened with a prior-to-exercise tolerance test. Also, in evaluating the amount of risk in their exercise programs, they should take into account such risk factors as the presence of coronary disease, high stress on the job, sedentary living, and cigarette smoking.

Healthy exercisers can also take heart at some other good news. Numerous studies by Ralph Paffenbarger and other noted researchers have identified exercise as a protective factor against coronary artery disease. In another recent report in the *Journal of the American Medical Association*, Dr. David S. Siscovick and others concluded that "high-intensity leisure time" activity—such as regular jogging at least three times a week—actually protects against primary cardiac arrest.

Specifically, Dr. Siscovick and his colleagues examined 163 cases of cardiac arrest in persons aged twenty-five to seventy-five years old, and comparing them to a control group, they determined that the risk of heart attack was 55 percent to 65 percent lower in persons with high-intensity leisure-time activity than in those without high-intensity activity.

The researchers acknowledged that vigorous physical activity has been associated in some studies with an enhanced risk of heart attack. But they believe that clinically healthy persons who engage in vigorous activity enjoy an overall reduction in their risk of heart attack.

Endurance exercise even seems to help animals avoid sudden death. One study of a group of dogs suggests that regular exercise can offer a degree of protection against fatal heart attacks. Interestingly, these dogs had previously been identified as being susceptible to sudden cardiac death. So it's possible that daily repetitive exercise may have provided a means of preventing sudden cardiac death among them, even though they were "high-risk patients."

In a Seattle study on humans, this view finds further support.

The researchers studied people who had suffered severe sudden cardiac arrest and then were resuscitated. They concluded that the people who were exercising regularly had a marked improvement in their chance of avoiding sudden death.

So to summarize, the weight of medical evidence tends to support the idea that exercise can place dangerous, additional stress on an already diseased and susceptible heart. On the other hand, in healthy individuals there is no evidence of any increased risk of sudden death from exercise. Moreover, the studies show that habitual, moderate exercise can decrease your risk of cardiovascular disease, and may offer some protection against sudden death.

Sudden death happens only rarely during sports. And when it does occur, congenital abnormalities or hardening of the arteries, or sometimes both, are usually to blame. As we've seen, arteriosclerosis is overall the largest cause of sports-related sudden death. For people at a high risk of developing cardiovascular disease, the possibility of sudden death may be great whether they exercise or not. So whatever their activity levels, these people should undergo treadmill stress testing and follow the recommendations that result from that test.

But now, how about you? Are you a person who is likely to be relatively free of risk of coronary artery disease? Or are you one of those people who is "susceptible" and therefore likely to develop heart trouble and suffer sudden death?

To answer these questions, let's turn now to the basic rules of risk for sudden death from heart disease.

CHAPTER FOUR

HOW TO REDUCE THE RISK OF HEART ATTACK AND SUDDEN DEATH BY UNDERSTANDING THE RULES OF RISK

Some people may point to an isolated instance of sudden death during exercise and then say, "This proves that exercise just isn't good for us!"

They may focus on the death of Jim Fixx or perhaps that of French marathoner Jacques Bussereau. Obviously, they say, such tragedies show we just weren't meant to run or jog.

Of course, these arguments ignore Fixx's and Bussereau's underlying heart problems. They also overlook the fact that such deaths are quite rare. Bussereau, for instance, was the first fatality among more than 100,000 runners who had participated in the New York marathon over the past fifteen years.

Since anyone can enter the New York marathon, even without medical screening, I'm surprised there has been only one death! This seems to suggest that marathon running may not be all that dangerous, or there would have been hundreds of deaths each year. After all, there are tens of thousands of people who now run marathons.

Still, the facts rarely get in the way. Through various kinds of twisted reasoning, the most radical critics will insist that exercise in modern society places an unnatural strain on the heart. Supposedly, it's virtually inevitable that average folks are just bound to crack under the pressure and do their bodies more harm than good.

Frankly, I think all this is unwarranted. In my opinion, we don't give our bodies enough credit. In our sedentary society, we don't even know the meaning of strenuous exercise. Most of us really have no idea what the human body can do with proper conditioning and nutrition. Your heart won't just give out automatically if you push yourself to the limit. To the contrary, the heart is an incredibly strong and efficient organ. With proper diet and conditioning, your body's potential can be pushed to unexpected heights.

Take the Tarahumara Indians in northern Mexico, for example. Their experience shows just how durable the heart can be. These Indians don't believe in taking it easy. In fact, social standing within the tribe often depends largely on their performance during a customary 75 to 100 mile ultra-marathon, during which they don't just run. During the entire event, they also must kick a small wooden ball in front of them!

Racing isn't like a weekend tennis game to these people. In fact, these races are such an important part of their lives that in their spare time the men think nothing of having a spontaneous practice race covering more than 50 miles! During a major race between competing groups within the tribe, they run continuously day and night through the mountains, sometimes for as long as forty-eight hours at a time, toward a goal often more than 150 miles away.

It is their endurance, not their speed, that makes these Indians so interesting to researchers. In one 28-mile "mini" race staged for a scientific study, the Indians were amused at the short distance. They regarded it as no more than child's play.

Over the course of the race, they averaged nearly six miles per hour, including breaks. That may not seem like an excessive pace, but remember: The race was conducted over extremely mountainous terrain. Researchers calculated that the amount of energy spent in completing the course at that speed surpassed what was humanly possible.

Yet, at the end of the race, the Indians stood calmly, breathing slowly and evenly, as the incredulous researchers examined them. Their blood pressure was even lower than when they had begun the race. Pulse rates when they crossed the finish line ranged from 120 to 150 beats per minute, compared with resting rates of 56 to 60 beats per minute.

But there's more: None of the Indians can recall a runner ever dropping out of a grueling race because of pain in his chest, or from shortness of breath that could be cardiac-related. Also, no one can recall a specific instance of sudden death, where one of the runners suddenly died in the course of a race from cardiac or circulatory problems. Finally, they have an extremely low level of arteriosclerosis.

Why do these Indians enjoy such protection from heart disease and sudden death? Is it genetics, or is something else at work?

Some natural selection, which would help to strengthen the gene pool of the community, may well be involved. For instance, the winners of the races become local celebrities. With this social prestige and popularity, they make very desirable mates. So, it's possible that over the years some sort of genetic tendency toward low heart disease and higher endurance has developed in the community.

Still, even though good genes may be a factor to some degree, they certainly don't tell the whole story. For one thing, scientific studies of this Indian community haven't confirmed that any "super gene" is involved. So we have to look elsewhere.

How about exercise? Of course, the Indian runners are superbly conditioned. From infancy, they learn to run almost as soon as they can walk. Even in childhood, they are accustomed to running everywhere by foot, racing through trails in the mountains. Everyone in the community, runner and nonrunner alike, gets around by walking. And because the Indians are farmers, virtually everyone is active in physically demanding agricultural work.

But even exercise can't provide the whole answer to the Indians' lack of coronary heart problems. Follow-up studies on the entire community of Indians, including those who tend to be more sedentary than the runners, have shown that there are *generally* low levels of arteriosclerosis.

So finally, we come to the food factor. In short, the community as a whole has a generally low-fat diet. Their meals consist primarily of corn and grain products, and only occasionally include meat. It's difficult if not impossible to find an overweight Tarahumara Indian. Moreover, their average adult cholesterol levels in one study were only 134, or far below that of the average American.

So it seems that the choice of lifestyle of these Indians, including a low-fat diet and a high level of cardiovascular fitness, has resulted in a community that is virtually immune to heart disease and sudden death. In contrast, common Western diets and lifestyles *do* promote heart disease.

It would appear, then, that we have something to learn from the experience in this Mexican community. Although they may not be as educationally or technologically advanced as many other Western groups, these Tarahumara Indians have shown us just how strong the heart can be if we give it half a chance.

As we've already seen in the first part of this chapter, heart attacks and sudden death are caused by coronary disease, not exercise. The best way to avoid heart attacks, then, is to minimize the chance of developing coronary disease. Medical research has revealed many factors that can increase the likelihood of developing coronary disease. We call these characteristics "risk factors."

While some risk factors can't be changed, there are some that we can help to minimize or avoid. Frequently, drugs or even surgery are needed to help. But for the most part, the risk factors can also be affected by changes in diet and lifestyle.

Now, let's take a closer look at the major risk factors for heart disease. These have been identified by the American Heart Association, and in many cases, I've expanded and adjusted them in light of the latest research. The eleven risk factors included here are not meant to be in any particular order or priority. You might want to compare the following information with the latest Coronary Risk Factor Charts we use at the Aerobics Center (see Appendix).

Risk Factor #1:   Family History and Heredity

Family history is one of those factors that you just can't do anything about. No amount of diet or exercise control is going to wipe out an inherited tendency to develop coronary disease. Certain cardiac disorders can be passed on from generation to generation, and may go unnoticed for many years. Then, they strike with lethal swiftness, as they did in the case of Jim Fixx. So, it's important that you know your family's history in order to get a truer profile of your own risk.

Of course, heredity can cut both ways. On the negative side, it can place you at increased risk if your ancestors have a history of dying at an early age from heart disease. Of course, it's important to identify exactly what is a "hereditary factor" and what isn't. You may not have too much to worry about if one of your relatives, who died of heart disease at an early age, was overweight, smoked excessively, and didn't exercise. His problem wasn't heredity at all; he was probably killed by environmental factors that won't affect you unless you have the same destructive lifestyle. On the other hand, what you *do* have to worry about is the relative who was lean and trim, didn't smoke, and exercised regularly—but who died before age fifty of heart disease. In this case, the problem is likely to be a hereditary predisposition, which may have been passed on to you.

Now, let's consider the positive side of things: Heredity can also offer some protection. We've all heard stories about people who smoke profusely, drink like a fish, and eat like there's no tomorrow—and then die at age ninety-five, perhaps as the result of a skiing accident. In fact, some people do seem to have a little extra something in their constitutional make-up to give them the ability to resist coronary disease better than others.

The Pima Indians of Arizona, for example, would ordinarily be considered prime candidates for coronary disease. They have the world's highest known rate of diabetes and one of the highest rates of obesity. Also, their diet consists almost entirely of high-fat "junk food." ("Heart Disease Found Low for Arizona Indian Tribe," *AMA News*, January 28, 1983.)

Yet, they have extremely low levels of harmful (LDL) cholesterol in their blood and very high levels of "good" or HDL cholesterol. And perhaps because of these facts, they contract heart disease seven times less frequently than the American white population. As a matter of fact, only 4 to 6 percent of those Pimas under sixty have abnormal electrocardiograms. This particular group has, in effect, developed a kind of genetic protection against coronary disease. Perhaps it's because they were lean and exercised vigorously and generally faced a tough, physically demanding existence in Southern Arizona's Gila River Valley until fifty years ago. Now, they lead a sedentary, impoverished life, and there is some question about how much longer their genetic protection will continue.

Unless you are a Pima Indian, however, don't count on an absence of heart disease in your family to shield you completely. Other studies suggest strongly that it's absolutely essential to watch your lifestyle and diet if you hope to minimize your risk of heart disease and sudden death.

For example, several studies of coronary disease among groups of natives in Pacific islands strongly suggest the potential dangers of a typical Western lifestyle. You see, even though their family and cultural backgrounds showed that these people were historically low in coronary disease, their communities showed increases in the number of coronary risk factors according to the extent to which they had adopted Western diet and other habits.

The classic example over the years has been the Japanese who moves to Hawaii or to the American West Coast. And now, with the "exporting" of Western culture to the islands of Japan, an alarming increase in deaths from cardiovascular disease is beginning to occur among that group. To help control and perhaps reverse this trend, our Institute for Aerobics Research collaborated with a group of businessmen and health professionals in Japan to establish the Nihon Aerobics Center near Tokyo. The Center opened in early 1985 and is expected to be a leader in the corporate wellness movement in the Far East. Such efforts should help prevent the onslaught of cardiovascular disease in those societies that accept Western diets and habits.

So, even though you can't change the fact that your ancestors had heart trouble, you can correct certain environmental factors such as a high-fat diet or sedentary living. In other words, you don't have to lose hope just because every male in your family had some degree of heart trouble in his early age. Instead, you should take extra care to reduce the other risk factors, wherever possible.

Risk Factor #2: Stressful Life and Personality

Chances are that you know some people who are compulsive, aggressive, or excessively achievement-oriented. They may show a sense of urgency about time and scheduling, and they may also seem to get hostile very easily at times. Commonly referred to as having the "Type A Personality," they are also seven times more likely to develop heart disease than their neighbors who have lower levels of stress. Cardiologists Ray Rosenman and Meyer Friedman have been the guiding lights in describing this stress-burdened type.

Other research has suggested that when we talk about a "stressful" life, we shouldn't limit ourselves to the obvious Type A's who are running around. There are also a group of people, recently labelled "Type C-Zone" personalities, who handle stress quite easily, without any of its debilitating effects. Such people have been described in some detail by Robert and Marilyn Kriegel in their fascinating book *The C Zone: Peak Performance Under Pressure.*

The big problem, though, is not with those who operate well under pressure. It's with the people who show signs of being unable to handle life's stresses. Sometimes, when people are dealt a devastating emotional blow, major physical problems can follow. For example, after a period of time, the cumulative effect of a stressful life can take its toll on the body in the form of heart disease.

According to the Holmes Life Change Score, a scale which reflects the impact of the major pressures in our lives, the most stressful events one can face include the death of a spouse, divorce, marital separation, detention in jail or other institution, and death of a close family member. Often, heart attacks are known to follow such stressful events. Learning how to deal better with life's stresses will definitely improve your probability of living longer.

We've had a number of experiences at the Cooper Clinic that show the effects of stress on people. About thirteen years ago, a man came to the Clinic after a heart attack at age thirty-nine. As he started exercising, restricting his diet and losing weight, he became very enthusiastic about his rehabilitation program.

For thirteen years he did extremely well; he was running 40 to 50 miles per week, with no heart symptoms or other problems. But in March 1983, when he came in for his annual examination, we noticed that his electrocardiogram during treadmill stress testing was grossly abnormal. During the previous tests, it had always been normal.

As a result, we altered his program a bit by revising his diet, weight, and exercise for a period of four months. When he returned after the four months were up, we put him back on the treadmill. Unfortunately, we found that the results were even worse than before.

Because of this "serial" change in his ECG, I suggested that he have a coronary arteriogram. The arteriogram, you'll recall, involves injection of a dye into the coronary arteries, followed by an X-ray procedure to determine whether they have been clogged by arteriosclerosis. The results were so bad that I recommended bypass surgery.

He recovered quickly from the bypass operation. In fact, he was discharged from the hospital after only five days, and two weeks after surgery he was able to walk and jog his first mile. The next month he walked and jogged a total of 146 miles—just six weeks from the time of his bypass surgery. Since then, he has worked up to the outstanding time of twenty-six minutes on the Balke treadmill test, just a bit shy of his all-time record of twenty-seven minutes and five seconds.

We really aren't certain what caused the sudden acceleration of this man's arteriosclerosis after nearly thirteen years of stability. But there were major changes in his life, stressful events that may have accelerated his heart problem.

Shortly before he came in for his examination in March 1983, he had divorced his wife of many years. As a result of the divorce, he left his home and seven children and moved out to a place of his own. He also changed his eating habits because he had to fix some of his own meals and eat in restaurants. And if those things weren't stressful enough, his business started going sour at about the same time.

It may be impossible to implicate stress alone as contributing toward arteriosclerosis in this case, but I suspect it played a key role. The effects of strong emotions are difficult to pinpoint because people who are in stressful situations such as this often tend to pursue unhealthy habits in other aspects of their lives. Often, they eat too much, or they change their diet to "fast foods" or meals that are high in saturated fats; they may also smoke or drink more than usual. In short, they just let themselves go.

But in many other cases, stress has been isolated as a major risk factor. A panel of the National Heart, Lung, and Blood Institute concluded that Type A behavior may increase the risk of coronary heart disease as much as high blood pressure, smoking, and high cholesterol levels.

There *are* things that you can do, however, if you are having problems associated with stress. In one recent study, heart attack victims with Type A behavior were given routine counseling, including suggestions about diet and exercise. Some victims, however, received suggestions on how to alter their Type A behavior. After one year, the researchers found that heart attacks and cardiovascular deaths were noticeably fewer in the group that had received behavioral counseling. In those patients who *did* suffer another heart attack, including those who died suddenly, researchers found that their attack immediately followed an emotional crisis, excessive exercise, or a fatty meal.

So, if you have a stress-oriented personality or the classic Type A variety, there is increasing evidence that you can alter the effects of these characteristics by voluntarily changing your lifestyle.

Another way to counter stress is to go the prescription route. One group of West German physicians has noted that beta-blockers—drugs commonly used to treat hypertension—can mitigate Type A behavior to diminish some of the more worrisome symptoms. An advantage of these drugs is that they do not have the typical side effects of sedatives or tranquilizers, such as drowsiness. Rather, most patients using beta-blockers are alert. It's possible, then, that certain drugs may be a possible alternative for persons at a high level of risk who can't seem to handle their stress through behavior modification.

But I always recommend a drug-free approach if that's at all possible. One of the best therapies for stressful personalities, routine exercise, may involve only a slight change in lifestyle. Exercise has been shown in many studies to act as a natural tranquilizer. Aside from feeling physically "spent" after dissipating frustrations through exercise, there's also a chemical reaction within our bodies. When we exercise, we release into our system hormones known as "endorphins," morphine-like substances that lower levels of pain and stress and make you feel "high." In this way, regular aerobic exercise can help relieve pent-up stress within your body and can enable you to keep it to manageable levels.

Risk Factor #3: High Blood Pressure, or Hypertension

When your blood pressure rises, damage to artery walls occurs and creates the sites where cholesterol can be deposited. There, it can form the plaques that develop into arteriosclerosis. The higher the blood pressure, and the more cholesterol in the blood, the faster these plaques will develop. Studies have shown that hypertensive patients are twice as likely to have heart attacks as people with normal blood pressure; six times more likely to have heart failure; and four times as likely to have strokes. (See *Nutrition & Health News*, Vol. II, No. 1; Fall, 1984.)

Adults are said to have elevated blood pressure, or hypertension, when their pressure exceeds 140 over 90. The higher your blood pressure is above this level, the greater your risk of cardiovascular disease.

At this mild stage, doctors may recommend only that their patients limit the amount of salt in their diets, shed excess pounds, stop smoking, and exercise.

As a matter of fact, according to a report in the *American Journal of Medicine* in 1984 (Vol. 77, p. 785), aerobic exercise *alone* has a beneficial effect on lowering blood pressure. In this study, 105 hypertensive patients began a graded exercise program, beginning with walking one mile a day and gradually escalating the activity level to two miles of jogging each day. The blood pressure of these patients was evaluated before exercise training and again three months after the participants were able to run 2 miles a day.

Even though half were receiving antihypertensive drug therapy at the beginning of the study, virtually all of the patients lowered their blood pressure. For the fifty-eight who were not receiving medication at the beginning of the study, diastolic pressure (blood pressure when the heart dilates) fell by fifteen points. In those who were on medication, mean diastolic blood pressure fell twenty points. Twenty-four of these patients were able to stop their medication altogether, and fourteen decreased their dose or discontinued one of their antihypertensive drugs.

Interestingly, the improvements were all independent of weight change. Ten percent of the patients had no change in weight; 30 percent gained some weight; 60 percent lost weight. In fact, the decrease in blood pressure with exercise training was as great in those who gained as in those who lost weight! But the beneficial effects didn't last without exercise. Of fifteen patients who returned to a sedentary life for three to four months, ten had significant increases in blood pressure.

Because hypertension is a key risk factor, even such "mild" hypertension must be taken very seriously. But we really don't worry about treating blood pressure medically until we get consistent readings above 150 over 95. When pressure gets to these more elevated levels, physicians often treat it with one of some thirty drugs presently available for hypertension. The most common ones are beta-blockers and diuretics that reduce the heart rate and flush excess sodium from your system.

Having your blood pressure checked is such a quick and easy test that you should have it done regularly. We also encourage patients to take their blood pressure at home. Excellent monitoring kits are available for $50 to $100. Also, if drugs have been prescribed for you, don't stop using them simply because you no longer feel any symptoms. Continued treatment is essential to avoid possible heart attacks, strokes, or sudden death.

Risk Factor #4: High Cholesterol and Triglycerides

High cholesterol and triglyceride levels have long been associated with coronary disease caused by arteriosclerosis. And the evidence still continues to mount. The National Heart, Lung, and Blood Institute recently released a report which confirms that in people with high cholesterol, lowering the level of cholesterol decreases the risk of heart attacks.

If your cholesterol level is in the seventy-fifth to ninetieth percentile range for your age group (i.e., 75 to 90 percent of all the people in your age group have a lower cholesterol level than you do), then your overall risk of death from heart attacks is moderate. If your cholesterol is above the ninetieth percentile level for your age group, your risk is high. You can see the age-adjusted levels of moderate and high coronary risk for both total cholesterol and also the total cholesterol/HDL cholesterol ratios in the table below. The term "mg/dl" stands for milligrams per deciliter.

Levels of Cholesterol and the Total Cholesterol/HDL Ratio

Age	Moderate Risk (75–90%)		High Risk (over 90%)	
	Choles. (mg/dl)	Ratio	Choles. (mg/dl)	Ratio
2–19	170–185	4.9–6.0	>185	>6.0
20–29	200–220	5.2–6.4	>220	>6.4
30–39	220–240	5.7–6.9	>240	>6.9
40 and over	240–260	6.2–7.5	>260	>7.5

(The cholesterol levels are taken from Consensus Development Conference Statement, National Institutes of Health, December 10–12, 1984. The ratios come from studies by the Institute for Aerobics Research in Dallas, November 1984.)

With aggressive lowering of cholesterol, up to a 50 percent reduction in cardiac deaths is possible. The ultimate goal should be to have cholesterol levels at less than 180 mg/dl for adults under thirty years of age, and less than 200 mg/dl for adults over thirty. Remember too, that for every 1 percent change in your cholesterol, the risk of heart disease changes by 2 to 3 percent.

In our search for more precise ways to measure risk, we have found that there are types of cholesterol that influence your risk of having heart disease. For example, low density lipoproteins (LDL) contain large amounts of cholesterol and other fats and a small amount of protein. LDL delivers the cholesterol to cells for storage. High levels of LDL cholesterol in the blood are a major factor in the acceleration of arteriosclerosis.

High density lipoprotein (HDL) is another type, which, in contrast to LDL, contains a small amount of cholesterol and other fats and a large amount of protein. HDL is responsible for transporting cholesterol from the body's tissue to the liver, where it is excreted as bile. A high level of HDL indicates a *decreased* risk of coronary heart disease and arteriosclerosis.

A third type of blood lipid is very low density lipoprotein (VLDL). This substance contains more fat than protein and consists mainly of triglycerides, rather than cholesterol. A high level of VLDL is thought to be associated with progressive arteriosclerosis. That's why high levels of triglycerides, even with normal cholesterol readings, should be avoided. (See Scott Grundy, M.D., Ph.D., *Nutrition & Health News,* University of Texas Health Science Center at Dallas, Vol. 2, No. 1, Fall 1984.)

At the Cooper Clinic, we have concluded that the ratio of total cholesterol to HDL cholesterol is a good predictor of a person's risk of coronary arteriosclerosis. That is, the lower the total cholesterol/HDL ratio, the lower the coronary risk. In several independent studies, this ratio of total cholesterol to HDL has alone correctly identified patients with coronary heart disease.

The famous Framingham Heart Study, now in its thirty-fifth year, has been *the* study to tie various risk factors to cardiovascular disease. One of the most important contributions of this National Heart, Lung, and Blood Institute-sponsored study has been linking the risk of cardiovascular disease to the level and kind of cholesterol in a person's blood. Framingham's director, Dr. William P. Castelli, recently said that the ratio of total cholesterol to HDL cholesterol in a person's blood is the single best predictor of a future heart attack. (See *The New York Times,* January 8, 1985.)

Lately, additional research has shed even more light on this HDL component. Now, we see that the HDL levels can be raised through lifestyle changes. In particular, routine exercise has been shown to be effective in shifting the balance of cholesterol and increasing the HDLs.

Surprisingly, though, some other studies have shown that a moderate amount of alcohol taken daily can also raise the HDL levels. But a follow-up study found that alcohol consumption had absolutely no impact on the HDL level in people who exercised regularly, while it increased the level in nonexercisers. This has led some people to believe that "jogging three miles or drinking three beers a day" can offer some protection against arteriosclerosis. However, we're finding that this isn't necessarily so.

You see, to make things even more complicated, your HDLs can also be separated into parts. When you exercise regularly, you raise your level of a special kind of high density lipoprotein—HDL-2. It is this HDL-2 type of cholesterol that is believed to offer some protection against arteriosclerosis.

On the other hand, when you drink alcohol in moderate amounts, you raise a subcomponent of your HDLs known as HDL-3. So far, studies have not shown any conclusive benefit against arteriosclerosis from an increase in HDL-3 level. It is true that some studies suggest a relationship between moderate use of alcohol and a decreased risk of coronary disease. Even so, there's no evidence that moderate alcohol consumption gives us the same long-term health benefits as does exercise. (For more on this, see Dr. William Haskell's article in the March 29, 1984 issue of the *New England Journal of Medicine.*)

As I see it, alcohol should never be considered as an alternative to exercise in promoting cardiovascular health. The negative effects on our health from drinking even moderate amounts of alcohol over a period of time will probably do far more harm than good.

Also, recent research indicates that a low level of HDLs may be related to cigarette smoking or the use of anabolic steroids. So stay away from them!

Now for another brief word on triglycerides. These fatty substances in the blood—which, you may recall, are the major constituents of VLDL—have a less clear connection to heart disease than does cholesterol. Numerous studies have shown us that high levels of triglycerides are strongly associated with coronary disease, particularly in conjunction with elevated cholesterol levels. It has also been shown that reducing triglyceride levels can reduce the rate of progression of arteriosclerosis. But many researchers still hesitate to recommend treatment for people with elevated triglycerides if they are otherwise healthy.

Triglyceride levels over a reading of 120 are generally considered excessive, though once again I'm a bit more careful. I prefer the level to be below 100.

Risk Factor #5:   Diabetes or High Levels of Glucose

Elevated glucose, or blood sugar, levels, such as those found in diabetics, have been related to a two- to three-fold increase in the number of deaths from coronary heart disease, as well as to nonfatal heart attacks. Cardiovascular disease is the leading cause of death in people with diabetes.

In diabetes, the patient is unable to burn up sugar because of an inadequate production of insulin by the pancreas. If an individual requires insulin to control diabetes, no insulin is being secreted by the body. In some cases, though, a form of diabetes occurs among adults when the pancreas can produce some but not enough insulin to meet the body's needs.

Your physician will usually confirm a diagnosis of diabetes by determining the blood sugar level in your body after a fourteen-hour fast. If that's inconclusive, then a two-hour test will be given after you've consumed a large amount of sugar.

Once diabetes has been diagnosed, diet is the main way to treat either type. In 80 to 90 percent of patients with adult-onset diabetes, diet and exercise can control the problem, particularly if the patient is overweight. More severe cases may require medication along with diet and exercise. Other research on patients with diabetes has revealed that exercise can actually decrease the amount of insulin a person requires; in effect, physical activity makes the body more responsive to the insulin that is produced. (See Philip Raskin's report in *Nutrition & Health News,* University of Texas Health Science Center at Dallas, Vol. II, No. 1, Fall 1984.)

To sum up, then, people with high levels of glucose are in distinct danger of developing diabetes. In addition to diet control, exercise has been shown to reduce certain other factors, such as excess body fat around or above the waist, that have been associated with diabetes.

Risk Factor #6:   Diet Rich in Fats and Cholesterol

For years, people refused to see the connection between the amount of cholesterol in their blood and the amount of cholesterol they eat in their food. Now, however, the evidence is overwhelming that a diet high in cholesterol and fats leads to elevated blood cholesterol levels. Over a long period of time, such a diet increases the risk of coronary disease.

In fact, most people who have heart attacks usually have at least mildly high blood cholesterol. As a result, greater numbers of doctors are pointing to diet as a major part of the problem—as well as part of the solution. In other words, a major approach to treatment is to go on a low-fat diet. Of course, diet alone may not be effective in severe cases of elevated cholesterol; in those situations, drugs must be used. But in mild cases, controlling what you eat is often the preferred first step of treatment.

Some interesting and provocative information has come from Nathan Pritikin's research into the effects of a very low-fat, low-cholesterol diet. His diet is roughly 80 percent complex carbohydrates, 10 percent fat, 10 percent protein, and less than 100 milligrams of cholesterol per day. Although it's a difficult program to follow for prolonged periods, researchers have observed marked reductions in total cholesterol, at least initially. Due to the high amounts of complex carbohydrates recommended by Pritikin, however, a person on this diet may well see a temporary elevation in the triglyceride levels.

Although it's still a highly controversial diet, Pritikin's approach does have a role in the management of patients with severe cholesterol problems, especially if they don't respond to routine dietary changes, weight loss, and exercise. In a number of cases in my own practice, before I've placed my own patients on medications to control an unresponsive, abnormally high cholesterol level, I've used the Pritikin diet with reasonable success.

Another interesting study has shown that arteriosclerosis can be affected not only by *what* we eat, but also by *when* we eat. You see, the peak time for digestion occurs about seven hours after consuming a heavy meal. This means that most of us are fast asleep when our gastric juices are doing the most work. The trouble with this is that we are loading fats and cholesterol into our bloodstreams at precisely the time when our body's metabolism has slowed down—and when it's least able to dispose of fats properly.

As a result, clots can form more easily, and that may result in stroke, heart attack, or sudden death. The researcher in the above study noted that in the Framingham report on coronary disease, more than half of the heart attacks occurred between 11 P.M. and 6 A.M., or the time when most of us are sound asleep. Also, heart attacks have often been found to follow an emotional, stressful event or a recent heavy, fatty meal.

In order to combat arteriosclerosis by reducing this risk factor, the American Heart Association recommends that people:

- Maintain an ideal weight. You should avoid becoming overweight by limiting your diet to one that excludes high-fat foods. Combine this diet with a program of regular endurance-type exercise, which has been shown to increase the proportion of HDL cholesterol.
- Reduce total fat in your diet to no more than 30 percent of the total amount of calories. The average for most people is now about 40 percent.
- Reduce the saturated fat in your diet to no more than 10 percent of the total calories (this includes fat from marbled meat, whole dairy products, animal fats such as butter, lard, and chicken fat, and vegetable oils such as coconut oil, palm oil, cocoa, hydrogenated margarine, and shortenings). Currently, most people ingest about 17 percent of their calories in saturated fats.
- Reduce consumption of cholesterol to a maximum of 300 milligrams per day, as opposed to the 500 to 550 milligrams that is commonly found in our diets. In particular, avoid egg yolks and

organ meats such as liver and kidney; limit high-cholesterol seafood such as squid and shrimp.

- Substitute polyunsaturated fats (corn, soybean, and safflower oils) and monosaturated fats (olive oil, peanut oil) for saturated fats. But levels of these should not exceed five percent of total daily caloric intake.
- Increase complex carbohydrates, including those found in vegetables, beans, grains, and cereals, to 50 to 55 percent of your daily calorie consumption. These substances also add fiber to the diet, which is believed to help lower the level of cholesterol in the blood.

With regard to this last point, diets high in fiber provide bulk, which helps to reduce the amount of cholesterol that is absorbed into the body. Some researchers believe, though, that some types of fiber may be more beneficial than others.

One study has shown that oat bran and dried beans are particularly effective in controlling cholesterol levels. According to this particular report, these foods contain "water-soluble fiber," as opposed to water-insoluble fiber. The insoluble fiber foods, which include such products as wheat bran, whole grains, fruits, and vegetables, tend to absorb water, increase bulk, and aid regularity. They are associated with a decreased risk of colon cancer, but they may not be as effective in lowering levels of cholesterol in your blood. So it's important to eat water-soluble fiber foods as well.

One issue that continues to generate controversy is whether or not coffee raises the level of cholesterol. In what can only be considered as bad news for the millions of people who enjoy coffee with breakfast, researchers in Norway recently found that coffee consumption *does* raise the cholesterol level. As a result, some researchers have said that drinking coffee in excess of nine cups a day may cause as much as a twofold rise in the risk of coronary disease.

But it's necessary to include a few qualifications here: The coffee preparation in Norway is different than it is in our country. They boil rather than brew their coffee, and 80 percent is consumed "straight," without any additives like milk. Other studies fail to support any increased risk of coronary disease with coffee consumption, particularly when it's taken in moderation and without an accompanying cigarette. (See the *New England Journal of Medicine,* Vol. 308, p. 1454, June 16, 1983.)

Risk Factor #7:　Inactivity and Sedentary Living Habits

While diet can be an important factor in determining the levels of cholesterol in your body, exercise is also a very important fat-affecting factor. For years, studies have confirmed that people who are inactive often have a higher level of cholesterol. As we have seen, it is generally their level of LDLs which is higher, a fact which leads to an increased risk of arteriosclerosis.

Some recent studies have shown that aerobic exercise can play a significant role in shifting the balance of HDL and LDL cholesterol in the body. In one report on the relationship of diet to HDL levels in marathoners, joggers, and sedentary men, diet was found not to be as significant as the amount of activity in which the men engaged. Also, the total distance run by the men was the best predictor of the proportion of HDL to total cholesterol. Overall, the study found that total cholesterol levels were lower in the distance runners, and their proportion of HDL cholesterol was greater. This conclusion again demonstrates a protective effect of distance running.

People who have led a sedentary life can help change their coronary risk profile by beginning to participate regularly in an endurance sport. In one group of sedentary men, several agreed to run regularly over a period of time to see if there would be any effect on their blood cholesterol levels. Then they were compared with some less active colleagues.

As it turned out, after one year of running the active group showed significantly lower overall cholesterol. And it didn't take a great deal to raise their HDL levels noticeably. Those runners who ran up to 15 miles a week regularly had a much higher proportion of HDL cholesterol than the control group. Clearly, you don't have to be a marathoner to get your blood in proper balance!

If the marked decrease in deaths from coronary heart disease in the past fifteen years is in any way related to the fitness exercise boom, it's most likely the result of an elevation in the HDLs. Furthermore, after bypass surgery, a worsening in coronary disease may be dependent upon a person's HDL levels as well.

In a ten-year study of eighty-two patients following coronary artery bypass surgery, those who had problems had high levels of

VLDL and LDL, and low levels of HDL. In fact, the level of HDL cholesterol was one of the major factors that distinguished between the two groups. So, exercise-induced elevations of HDL may be the best thing a coronary artery bypass patient can do to prevent further progression of the disease. (See the *New England Journal of Medicine*, pp. 1329–1332, November 22, 1984.)

Risk Factor #8:   Cigarette Smoking

The adverse effects of cigarette smoking on your health are now well documented. Smokers are far more likely to develop coronary disease than nonsmokers, and the death rate from coronary disease— including sudden death—is far higher in smokers. In fact, cigarette smoking is one of the three most important risk factors, along with hypertension and an elevated level of cholesterol. Yet many people continue to smoke because they don't notice any physical problems. Many smokers have told me, "The damage is already done, so there's no point in quitting now!"

Not only is that a dangerous attitude, but it's also untrue. Regardless of your age, there is a remarkable improvement in your health when you stop smoking. The *Journal of the American Medical Association* reported a study in 1984 that considered whether cigarette smoking retained its adverse effects on survival in an elderly population. Current cigarette smokers had a risk of death from coronary heart disease that was 59 percent higher than nonsmokers, ex-smokers, or cigar or pipe smokers. But there was good news along with the bad: The excess risk declined within one to five years after they stopped smoking. So elderly smokers should always be encouraged to quit!

The same principle applies to younger people. An Oslo study, reported in the December 12, 1981 issue of the British medical journal *Lancet*, followed 1232 healthy men, forty to forty-nine years of age, for five years. The purpose was to see if lowering the blood cholesterol and cessation of smoking could reduce the incidence of coronary heart disease. Men were admitted to the study if they had normal blood pressure, had cholesterol readings between 290 and 380 milligrams, and smoked cigarettes.

Those who tried to change their risk factors were only mildly successful: On average, they dropped their cholesterol by 13 percent;

25 percent stopped smoking; and 45 percent decreased the number of cigarettes smoked daily. But even with these moderate changes, at the end of the five years the results were rather dramatic: Deaths from heart attacks and sudden deaths in general were 47 percent lower in the intervention group than in the controls! As you can see, it doesn't take major changes in lifestyle or habits to see remarkable improvements in health.

It does take some time to undo the damage of a long-term smoking habit. But after a period of time, smokers who break the habit may reduce their risk of developing or dying from coronary artery disease to the same level as nonsmokers. As we've already seen, researchers have found that smokers who quit reduce their risk somewhat after one to five years of nonsmoking.

But don't make the mistake of believing that if you smoke a cigarette low in nicotine, you'll be less affected by the nicotine. Unfortunately, such conclusions, as advertised in some commercials, are based on the results of nicotine studies that used measurements made by *smoking machines*. Machines, however, don't smoke like people do. Actual blood concentrations were measured in 272 subjects smoking various brands of cigarettes, according to a 1983 report in the *New England Journal of Medicine*. There, the investigators didn't find that smokers of low-nicotine cigarettes consumed any less nicotine.

Another study, reported in the *Journal of the American Medical Association* in 1983, showed that smoking cigarettes was a potent risk factor in decreasing blood flow to the brain. Probably, this enhanced cerebral arteriosclerosis. If so, this finding suggests an increased risk for strokes among smokers.

Even smokers with heart-related chest pain benefit when they stop smoking. Those who quit for just a brief period have been found to decrease their heart rates and improve their electrocardiogram test results.

The damage of smoking goes further than just increasing the risk of coronary disease—it also interferes with treatment. Angina patients who smoked were found to be less responsive to drug treatment for their chest pains than nonsmokers. But, again, this was not a permanent condition. When smoking patients ceased smoking for just one month, their episodes of angina came less frequently. Also, the painkilling drugs prescribed to them were more effective.

Over the years, a multitude of different approaches have been used to help people break the cigarette smoking habit—with variable degrees of success. Recently, a 2-milligram nicotine chewing gum has been added to the list of options. In one study presented in the *Journal of the American Medical Association* in 1984, 29 percent of those who used this gum as a part of group therapy stopped smoking. In contrast, only 16 percent who were treated with a placebo gave up smoking. Apparently, a combination of nicotine gum and group therapy can be of some help in improving the success rates of stopping smoking.

Risk Factor #9: Obesity

Ordinarily, people think of "obese" as referring to someone who is grossly overweight. But in considering good health, if you are even moderately above your ideal weight, you are "obese" in terms of increasing your risk of developing coronary disease.

For some time, researchers have seen the association between obesity and coronary disease. But many have thought that the disease was brought on by other factors such as hypertension, high levels of cholesterol and triglycerides, and high levels of blood sugar. In recent studies, however, there are strong indications that—even if your blood pressure is normal, and other risk factors are in line—just being overweight increases your risk of developing coronary disease.

A person's percentage of body fat, which is the best way to determine your ideal weight, can be determined either by the use of skin caliper measurements or by hydrostatic (underwater) weighing. The acceptable percentages of body fat for various age groups are as follows:

Acceptable Percentages of Body Fat

	Men		Women	
Age	Acceptable	Ideal	Acceptable	Ideal
Under 30	13.0	9.0	18.0	16.0
30–39	16.5	12.5	20.0	18.0
40–49	19.0	15.0	23.5	18.5
50–59	20.5	16.5	26.5	21.5
Over 60	20.5	16.5	27.5	22.5

These acceptable standards have been developed from the data collected on more than 30,000 patients involved in the Aerobics Center longitudinal research study.

Risk Factor #10:   Abnormal Resting Electrocardiogram

An electrocardiogram (ECG) is a test that measures the performance of your heart electrically. A person who shows an abnormal reading while at rest may be considered a high risk for coronary disease. The resting ECG abnormality most commonly associated with an increased risk of developing coronary disease is called "left ventricular hypertrophy," or enlargement involving a disproportionate increase in the size of one chamber of the heart.

Often, though, resting ECGs that appear normal may actually be masking some underlying disease that can only be detected when high demand is placed on the heart. To find these underlying heart problems, ECGs must be taken while people are exercising vigorously, such as on a treadmill. We'll see how this works when we explore treadmill stress testing in later chapters.

Risk Factor #11:   Oral Contraceptives

The main problem with birth control pills is that they generally contain some combination of estrogen and progesterone. The risk of cardiovascular disease from oral contraceptives is thought to be related both to the estrogen and to the potency of the progesterone. High-potency combinations of progesterone have in many studies been associated with high levels of LDL cholesterol and low levels of HDL cholesterol. And of course, high LDL and low HDL have been linked to an increased risk of coronary heart disease.

But you can minimize this pill problem. For instance, you might lower the dosage. Birth control pills containing 30 to 35 micrograms of estrogen are seemingly as effective in preventing pregnancy as are the 50-microgram pills. Serious cardiovascular problems are usually associated with pills that have an estrogen level of more than 50 micrograms. Also, there are several compounds available that have low-potency progesterone, yet are still recognized as effective contraceptives.

But there are some disadvantages of low-potency oral contraceptives that must be taken into account. Women who use these drugs do lower their risk of cardiovascular disease. At the same time, they have higher rates of spotting, breakthrough bleeding, and pregnancy. Only you in consultation with your physician can make the best decision for your situation.

Aside from the amount of estrogen and progesterone in the birth control pills, researchers say that cardiovascular problems are most frequent in women who use oral contraceptives and are over the age of thirty-five, who smoke heavily, or who have other coronary risk factors. Obviously, there's nothing you can do about your age. But if you decide to continue to use oral contraceptives, you can lower their overall risk of causing heart disease and sudden death by quitting smoking and by reducing other risk factors where possible.

Here's another point where moderate exercise has been shown to help. While some women using oral contraceptives have been shown to develop blood clots, a recent report says that this problem can be reduced or eliminated if they exercise. An enzyme called plasmin, which is found naturally in the walls of arteries, breaks down clots before they can do any serious damage.

In the study, women who developed blood clots while taking oral contraceptives showed a reduced plasmin level. Moderate exercise, however, has shown some protection. In a group that exercised three times a week for thirty to forty-five minutes at a time, the plasmin levels increased between 50 and 250 percent.

Continuing the use of estrogens after menopause may have some beneficial effects in reducing the problem with heart disease. But again, there is a trade-off. Postmenopausal estrogens are clearly related to an increased risk of some types of cancers, such as cancer of the uterus. The relationship between estrogen therapy and other types of cancer is not as clear.

Those risk factors that are associated with heart attacks and sudden death are by no means written in concrete in your life. There are a host of ways you can reduce the possibility of death during exercise or even while you're sitting quietly in your home. Simple changes in the way you live your daily life can greatly increase your chances to live a longer, healthier life.

As we saw with the Tarahumara racers at the beginning of this chapter, a properly conditioned heart is capable of remarkable strength and endurance when it is unfettered by coronary disease.

Yet our lifestyles—what we do and what we eat—tend to work against this natural ability. We tend to gravitate toward lives that place very few demands on our bodies. As a result, our level of conditioning frequently falls to the extremely low levels of a sedentary existence.

But you *can* change your lifestyle today and, in doing so, decrease your risk of coronary disease. One of the best and most enjoyable ways, as we'll see in the next two chapters, is to embark on a *safe* aerobic exercise program.

CHAPTER FIVE

THE FUNDAMENTALS OF EFFECTIVE EXERCISE— WITH A WARNING ABOUT THE GREAT COOL-DOWN DANGER

"Rejoice, we conquer!" gasped Pheidippides, perhaps the most acclaimed endurance athlete of all time. And with these words, he fell down dead.

He had just run from the Plain of Marathon to Athens, a distance of more than 26 miles, to announce the victory of the Greeks over the Persians in 490 B.C.

Through the ages this story has been related as an example of selfless patriotism. Countless school children have heard the tale and assumed that his death resulted from the supreme physical effort he had made. Or perhaps his stout runner's heart burst with sheer joy after he reported the glorious news of triumph to the Athenian citizens. The marathon race, which was never part of the ancient games, has been added to the modern Olympics in memory of Pheidippides' effort.

But it's the factual rather than the fanciful cause of Pheidippides' sudden death that fascinates me. I can only speculate that he was chosen as the bearer of such important news because he was noted for his running ability. So, I think it's reasonable to assume that this first marathon runner was a man who was in excellent physical condition and who probably had a reputation for running swiftly over long distances. Yet he was struck down by sudden death. Why?

In the accounts we have of this ancient event, one point stands out above the rest: Pheidippides didn't die until *after* he had stopped running. In other words, he expired during the so-called "cool-down" phase of his athletic effort. This phenomenon of the "post-exercise peril" is to this day a major danger that's not fully understood. As we've seen, an inadequate cool-down may have been a factor in Jim Fixx's death. So this key phase of a workout is certainly something you should understand as you seek to build a safe personal exercise program.

In an attempt to find an explanation for the potentially fatal threat of the cool-down, some Harvard and Tufts University doctors recently conducted a study of ten healthy men between the ages of twenty-two and thirty-five. Each man was asked to sit on a stationary bicycle ergometer, an apparatus used to measure work performed by a group of muscles. Then, they were told to begin pedaling.

After three minutes, each man's blood pressure was recorded and a blood sample was taken. The resistance on the ergometer wheel of the bicycle was then increased so that the individual had to work harder. He continued to pedal for another three minutes, and then, once again, his blood pressure was measured and a blood sample drawn.

This pattern was repeated until the man was exhausted. At that point, the resistance on the bicycle wheel was released, and he was asked to pedal freely for a "cool-down" of two three-minute periods. The researchers continued to take blood pressure readings and blood samples during this cool-down phase.

The study revealed some interesting facts about the changes that take place in the body during such workouts. As the researchers had expected, the levels of two natural stimulants produced by the adrenal glands, epinephrine (also called adrenaline) and norepinephrine, increased in the blood during the most strenuous part of the exercise. Also, blood pressure went up during this phase.

But then, as the blood pressure dropped during the cool-down period, when the intensity of exercise was decreasing, the levels of epinephrine and norepinephrine *continued* to rise. Because these adrenal substances are natural heart stimulants, the researchers think they may have found the mechanism that triggers potentially dangerous, irregular heartbeats after strenuous exercise. In other words, the continued production by the body of natural stimulants may be a key to understanding how the heart can begin to beat out of control, and perhaps even lead to death.

The doctors speculated that the marked increase of norepineph-rine in particular may be a reflex effort to keep blood pressure at the maximum levels achieved during strenuous exercise. It takes a while for this natural "hyping-up" of the exerciser's body to slow down—a fact that has important implications for the safest way to end an endurance workout. In short, the body must be allowed to return *gradually* to its pre-exercise state.

"The worst possible strategy for exercise cessation would be to have the patient abruptly stop exercising and stand," the researchers concluded. "The best strategy would be for the work load to be diminished gradually and/or for the subject to rest supine after the exercise."

In short, anyone who stops vigorous exercise abruptly is endangering his heart—and may be flirting with sudden death. The circulatory system in a sense goes "out of balance" as the flow of blood slows down faster than the beating of the heart.

If you stop and stand still without reducing the level of your activity step by step, your blood pressure will drop. But the natural stimulants from the adrenal glands keep the heart beating at a high and inefficient rate. As a result, not enough blood gets to the heart, and ischemia of the heart, involving a lack of blood to the heart tissue, may result. If there is too little blood that gets through to the heart, sudden death may occur.

As we've already seen, this is what may have happened to Jim Fixx when he collapsed just after his run in northern Vermont. He came to rest with his head and heart above his legs. In this position, blood which had "pooled" in the legs and in the vessels below the waist could not get back to his heart.

In most cases, if a person collapses because of prolonged standing or an inadequate cool-down, he'll just fall flat to the ground and gravity will move the blood back to the heart and head. Then, he'll regain consciousness and probably recover rather quickly. But there's enough chance of a fatality in this situation for me to recommend strongly that every regular exerciser take special care to go through a proper cool-down phase after a workout.

So, what exactly constitutes a proper, safe cool-down procedure?

The basic, guiding principle is *never stop exercising suddenly.* The drop in blood pressure during the cool-down phase should take place gradually. That means you have to keep moving, swiftly at first, and then at a somewhat slower pace. Usually, if you're a runner, a steady, brisk walk will do the job. If you're a swimmer, you might continue to move your arms and legs in the water, perhaps in a treading motion or walk around in the shallow end of the pool.

If you're walking, move along at a pace of about two to three miles per hour and place your arms above your head if you start to feel light-headed. This keeps the blood pressure up and the blood circulating to your heart and head. Continue these movements for at least three to five minutes—and I prefer it to go for a longer rather than shorter period of time.

Above all, after you've completed the most vigorous phase of your workout, follow each of these all-important "don'ts":

• Don't stand still.
• Don't sit.
• Don't stand motionless while taking your pulse. When you check it, keep moving!
• Don't start talking and get distracted to the extent that you forget to keep moving. When you come to the end of your workout, your mind should automatically tell you, "Keep moving, keep moving, keep moving!"
• Don't come to a complete halt at a stoplight or stop sign. Obviously, you don't want to run out headlong into traffic—that could be more dangerous than an inadequate cool-down. But I do recommend that you continue to run in place or jog a short distance back and forth at the corner until the light changes or traffic clears.

If, after an all-out or competitive performance, you feel nausea or light-headedness during your cool-down, you may find you simply can't keep moving. In this case, it's a good idea to lie down flat on your back for a few minutes to let your body return more or less to normal. When you do this, your head should stay level with or below your feet. If you're in a gym, you might lie down on a mat, or when outdoors, you can stretch out on grass or a park bench and prop up your feet. By following this procedure, you'll be more likely to avoid a precipitous drop in blood pressure or some other abnormality that could cause you to lose consciousness or even die.

In my other books I discuss what constitutes proper aerobic exercise. But when safety is involved, there can never be too much of a good thing. So, in the next few pages, I want to give you a brief description from the ground up of the key features that should be present in the soundest, most effective aerobic programs.

First of all, let's get some basic definitions out of the way. The word "aerobic," you may recall, means living in air or utilizing oxygen. You're in an aerobic state when you sit in a chair and breathe normally because the amounts of oxygen that you're taking in and that your body is using are in balance.

As you begin to exercise, however, your body requires more oxygen. As a result, your rate of breathing increases, and your heart pumps faster to supply the extra oxygen. But as was the case when you were sitting, you can stay in an aerobic state during exercise as long as you maintain a balance between your intake of oxygen and your output of bodily energy. On the other hand, if you exercise too hard, you may become "anaerobic." That is, your body will begin to use more oxygen than you take in, and you'll quickly become exhausted.

So, aerobic exercises are those which are designed to increase your breathing and heart rates for a relatively long period of time, without disturbing the balance between your intake and use of oxygen. Running, swimming, cycling, cross-country skiing, dancing, and other such activities, if they are done at a less-than-maximum intensity over long distances or periods of time, tend to be aerobic. In contrast, sports like sprinting, which require sudden, excessive spurts of energy, are anaerobic.

We've discovered that aerobic exercise, done regularly over a period of weeks, can produce a "training effect." That is, this activity puts the body into better shape and increases an individual's capacity to do increasingly strenuous exercise. The results include a fitter cardiovascular system, the reduction of sedentary living and other risk factors, and greater protection from heart disease.

To produce the greatest benefit, a common approach is to use your "target heart rate," which is defined as 65 to 80 percent of your maximum heart rate. A healthy person can figure his target heart rate this way:

Step One: Find your resting heart rate by pressing your wrist with your middle two fingers and counting the number of beats per minute of your pulse. Practice until you are competent and consistent with this measurement.

Step Two: Determine your "predicted maximum heart rate" (PMHR). If you're a man and have been exercising regularly, this would be 205 minus one-half your age. If you're a woman or a totally unfit man—both of whom tend to have comparable PMHRs—it's 220 minus your age. So, if you're a forty-year-old woman, your PMHR would be 180, and if you're a physically fit man of the same age, it would be 185.

Step Three: Finally, figure your target heart rate *zone.* You do this by taking both 65 percent and 80 percent of your PMHR. So, if you're the forty-year-old woman mentioned above, you would multiply 0.65 times 180 for a lower range of 117, and 0.80 times 180, for the upper target heart rate of 144. Your zone would thus be 117 to 144.

When you've figured your target heart-rate zone, then you should choose an exercise which will enable you to get your heart up to that rate for at least twenty minutes a day, four times a week. If you can achieve this level of exercise, you'll quickly begin to experience the training effect that will improve your physical condition and the strength of your heart.

Contrary to the expectations of many, you don't have to exercise vigorously to get a good aerobic training effect. Dr. Steven Blair, director of epidemiology for our Institute for Aerobics Research, conducted a study on low-intensity exercise programs while he was at the University of South Carolina. He was able to show a highly significant improvement in aerobic fitness for young, healthy male subjects, who exercised at only 50 percent of their maximal performance for thirty to forty minutes, five days a week for ten weeks.

It's reasonable to believe that with longer-lasting exercise sessions at even lower heart rates, a significant training effect will occur. This means that walking can be an effective way to condition yourself aerobically, provided you do enough of it. I've recommended in previous books that you might work up to walking 3 miles in forty-five minutes, five days per week. Or you might run 2 miles in less than twenty minutes, four times per week.

Now, let me walk you through some of the practical steps you'll need to take to get started on your own personalized aerobic exercise program. First of all, some preliminary guidelines:

• *Pick an exercise you enjoy and are likely to continue.* One consideration is to choose the place where you will be exercising and to determine how easy it is to get there. Obviously, it doesn't make much sense to pick swimming if the nearest pool is twenty miles away and you only have forty-five minutes available for your workout.

Also, do you have the necessary skill to get the most out of the exercise? Or will you be limited in how much physical activity you can engage in because you're a beginner? For example, it could be difficult to get in a sufficient amount of aerobic activity if you're just learning how to ski or swim. You'll spend so much time working on your technique that you'll fail to get your heart rate up to a high enough level to achieve a training effect.

In addition, you'll have to consider whether your sport requires a partner or team. If so, how available are these other participants? Also, how expensive is the activity—within your price range or above it?

Finally, remember that several studies have shown greater adherence and fewer injuries in lower intensity programs, like walking, than with more vigorous programs. And the same end results can be achieved as with high intensity programs; it just takes longer.

• *Consider getting a medical check-up before you begin.* An exam is mandatory if you are over forty; are twenty pounds or more overweight; have a family history of premature heart disease; smoke; have high blood pressure; or have a high cholesterol count. No exam is complete without a treadmill stress test of the type we'll discuss later in this book.

• *If you feel any chest discomfort or other continuing pain after you begin to exercise, stop immediately and check with a doctor.* Pain or discomfort is always a signal that you should quit.

• *Progress slowly.* Don't push yourself into doing too much too soon. If you've been out of shape for years, you can't expect to get back into condition overnight.

Also, some commercial exercise programs require a physical fitness test in order to determine in which class you belong. This may or may not be a wise practice. Under proper supervision, such a test can have merit, but improperly administered, it can be dangerous.

In fact, if you're just starting out, I'd advise you against taking any all-out fitness test which pushes you to the limits of your endurance. The only exceptions would be if you've been exercising regularly for at least six weeks or if you're medically monitored while the test is being administered.

A good means of measuring whether or not you're pushing too hard during exercise is the "talk test." That is, see if you can continue to talk to people while you're in the process of exercising. If you become too breathless to speak, then you're "pushing too hard."

These, then, are the basic, preliminary guidelines you should keep in mind before you embark on an exercise program. After you actually get started, any safe, effective aerobic program you choose should include at least these four basic phases:

Phase #1: The Warm-Up

The first step in each of your exercise sessions should be the warm-up. I recommend that you spend at least three to five minutes stretching and getting your muscles warm. It's best to begin with undemanding exercises, such as swinging your arms and gently stretching your back, neck, and legs.

A favorite of mine, particularly if you have any problem with lower back pain, is the so-called "Williams" group of exercises. To do these, you lie flat on your back and then pull your left knee up to your chest and hold it there for a few seconds. Then, do the same with your right knee. Finally, pull both of your knees to your chest, hold them there for a few seconds, and return to the starting position. Then, begin again for a total of about five full cycles.

I usually finish off this group of exercises with a maneuver called the "pelvic tilt." This involves lying flat on my back and then flattening the small of my back against the floor and holding it there for a few seconds. This series of exercises can be done any time of the day by those with chronic low-back problems.

Next, you might move into a more vigorous warm-up, perhaps with some jumping jacks or running in place for thirty to sixty seconds. This helps you increase your heart rate and prepares you for the more strenuous aerobic phase of the workout. A proper warm-up may even decrease the "oxygen debt" reached during aerobic activity; in other words, you may find it increases your overall endurance. Also, the warm-up will help reduce muscular and skeletal injuries.

Let me give you an example of how omission of this warm-up

phase may have caused a problem. A woman who had been a participant in one of our programs for several months rushed late into her exercise class one cold winter day. The class had already done their basic stretching exercises, and they were starting with the more demanding aerobic phase. Instead of beginning by doing some slow stretching on her own, however, the woman started the more demanding jumping and dancing that the class was doing. She instantly felt something snap in one of her calves. Sharp pain immobilized her, and she had to be carried to a chair, where ice was applied to her leg.

Later, she learned she had torn her plantaris ligament. Consequently, she had to stay off her leg for a week and walk with a cane for some time after that. Eventually, her leg healed, of course. But even a few months after this incident, she still experienced some discomfort during exercise in her injured leg.

It's impossible to say definitely that an inadequate warm-up was responsible for her injury. But pulled or torn muscles and ligaments are much more common in an extremity that is cold and improperly warmed-up.

Another advantage of the warm-up is to prepare the cardiovascular system for exercise. Many studies have shown that in patients with heart disease, higher work loads can be achieved without angina or chest pain *if* a warm-up precedes the exercise. On the other hand, going from a resting state to an all-out performance on a treadmill can produce ECG abnormalities, even in people with no heart disease.

In short, it's foolish to risk injury because you get impatient to get right into your workout. Take it easy at the beginning, and your body will be better prepared to take some tough challenges later, when you engage in the more strenuous aerobic phase of your program.

Phase #2: Aerobic Exercise

This is the part of your program which is designed to raise your heart to that target level, which will be somewhere between 65 and 80 percent of its maximum. Remember: You're striving here to achieve a balance between oxygen intake and energy outflow, a state that will allow you to get the maximum increase in cardiovascular fitness. If you're exercising four times a week, you should devote at least twenty minutes per session to this aerobic phase. If you exercise three times a week, the minimum for each aerobic section should be thirty minutes.

The aerobic phase is the core of your physical fitness program. But as the old saying goes, you should "train, not strain." In other words, you must reach a plateau of heightened activity where you'll keep your heart rate within the "target heart rate zone" you determined a few pages back.

Finally, some runners, swimmers, and cyclers enjoy putting on an extra burst of speed at the end of this aerobic phase. This final sprint is sometimes called "kicking." If you do "kick in" at the end of a strenuous workout, you should pay attention to how your body responds. Is there any discomfort or pain anywhere in your body? If so, you may be overextending yourself. In the future, you should be content with an even pace throughout your workout. Irregular heartbeat activity is a way the heart may rebel. Frequently, I see such abnormalities during the final few seconds of a maximal performance treadmill test. They may or may not persist throughout recovery after the test.

In any case, after a "kick," it's a good idea to give yourself a more complete and lengthy cool-down than normal. You'll find that pampering your body a little at this stage can pay safety dividends in the long run.

Phase #3: The Cool-Down

My experience as well as the experience of others indicates that if a heart attack does occur during athletic activity, approximately half the time it will happen *following* vigorous exercise. That means the attack will hit you during the period when your body is just starting to cool down from a hard workout. So be sure you don't ignore this phase, at the end of a workout!

As I mentioned earlier, you should spend at least five minutes cooling down. And remember: Take longer if you've ended your aerobic phase in a final burst of speed. This means that you should keep walking and moving about until your heart rate drops to less than 120 beats per minute, or less than 100 if you are over fifty years of age. If the heart rate stays higher than these levels during the five-minute recovery, you should not exercise as vigorously or as long the next time out.

In fact, I use this heart rate response during recovery after exercise more than I do the maximal heart rate as a measure of whether the exercise is safe. The only exception is a cardiac patient who is involved in a rehabilitation program. In these cases, the individuals are given a maximum heart rate (as determined by the results of their stress tests) which can be achieved during exercise. Staying at or below this rate must be rigidly enforced by the use of various monitoring techniques.

Most important of all, stay aware of your body and its reactions at all times during this cool-down phase. If you feel a little "funny" at any point during the cool-down, you may want to have your doctor check you out. In any case, don't sit down to rest until you've cooled down adequately in accordance with the guidelines I've given you.

Phase #4:   Calisthenics and Weight Training

This phase, which should normally be done at the end of your workout or on a day when you're not involved in your main aerobic activity, involves doing special exercises to build up your muscles. By strengthening your muscles, you'll toughen your body and minimize the danger of injury during the aerobic period of your program. Common exercises to achieve the goals of this phase include basic muscle-strengthening calisthenics such as push-ups, chin-ups, leg-lifts, and various types of standard weight-lifting. Also, you may want to use some of the other equipment now available, such as the Universal Gym or the Nautilus.

I would encourage you *not* to do these exercises before your aerobic phase because you'll tend to build up the "oxygen debt" before you enter your aerobic phase. That is, you'll wear yourself out and may be too exhausted at the beginning of your workout to get the greatest benefits from the endurance activity you've chosen. If you have any underlying heart disease, this extra burden you'll be putting on your system could even be dangerous.

But generally speaking, it's safe to follow a systematic, moderately demanding calisthenics or weight-training program after your aerobic workout or on alternate days. I suggest that you try doing these special, strength-building exercises a minimum of ten minutes a day, three times a week.

In addition to the classic strength-enhancing programs, some joggers these days are conditioning their upper bodies with Heavy Hands. These are two small weights of three to five pounds each. You hold one in each hand during your aerobic workout and move them about in various ways to strengthen your arms, shoulders, chest, back, and legs. However, running with weights in the hands may cause symptoms in patients with underlying cardiovascular problems.

The benefit of carrying this extra weight is twofold: First of all, it increases the intensity of your workout, and this enhances the aerobic training effect of a workout. Also, as I've said, the small weights condition your arms, upper body, and legs.

Our research institute at the Aerobics Center recently completed a ten-week study on the aerobic and strength effect of exercising with a heavy rope. These weighted ropes varied from two and one-half to six pounds and were used in an interval training program.

Four times per week, the subjects would skip rope for one minute; each of these sessions was followed by a one-minute rest. The work-rest cycle continued for a total of twenty-two minutes. Substantial improvement was seen in both the aerobic capacity and the strength of the upper extremities, according to researcher Dr. Jill Upton. In fact, the improvement was comparable to what I've documented in previous books under the subject of circuit weight training.

Finally, let me say a few words about motivation. If you hope to continue exercising on a regular basis for the rest of your life, it's essential to learn how to keep your interest level high. One way is to compete against yourself, such as by keeping records of your progress. You might take your measurements, weigh yourself, and note improvements in your time and distance.

Another, more comprehensive way to chart your progress is to find a way to follow a scientifically proven approach to measuring aerobic fitness. In my previous book, *The Aerobics Program for Total Well-Being*, I outlined an aerobics points system that can assist you in measuring the amount of energy you expend in performing various exercises for given periods of time and given distances. Many of my patients and readers have discovered that the point system, or some similar method, can be a good way to monitor the effectiveness of their program and to answer that nagging question, "Am I exercising enough?"

In addition to watching your own progress, you may find that you stick to a program more consistently if you work out in a class or with a partner. Sometimes, the idea that you've invested money in an exercise program, whether for equipment or classes, can keep you going for a while.

As for me, I say use any technique that suits you—so long as it keeps you exercising. If you can keep at an aerobics program for at least six weeks, and you're exercising three to four times a week during that period, I'm convinced you'll be less likely to give it up. You'll begin to notice such a change in your physical and emotional well-being that you'll probably be ready to commit yourself for the rest of your life.

But at this point, if you haven't already embarked on an endurance exercise program, you may be wondering about the specifics of particular aerobics exercises. For example, what are the benefits of swimming, as opposed to running, cycling, or aerobic dancing? What is the best activity for you?

To answer these and similar questions, let's examine some of the most popular aerobic sports in more detail.

CHAPTER SIX

WHICH AEROBIC EXERCISE IS RIGHT FOR YOU? A SURVEY OF SAFE AND EFFECTIVE ALTERNATIVES

I've called this book *Running Without Fear,* but it could just as easily be entitled, *Exercising Without Fear.* There are a number of excellent, safe ways to get into tip-top shape, and I now want to explore seven of the most popular in some detail. If you pursue them intelligently, you'll be less likely to suffer a sports injury. And most important of all, you'll lower your coronary risk factors and reduce the likelihood of developing heart disease.

Cross-Country Skiing

This sport is the most strenuous of all the aerobic activities. I rank it number one for several reasons: The most important is the fact that the most highly conditioned aerobic athletes in the world (i.e., those with the highest measured maximal oxygen consumption) are the Scandinavian cross-country skiers. I'm sure that the reason for this is that cross-country skiing requires the use of several major muscle groups, including those of the legs, arms, and trunk. Some of the other top aerobic exercises only focus on one set of muscles, such as the legs. In addition, cross-country skiing is usually done at relatively high altitudes, puts more demands on the body because it has to be done out of doors in cold weather, and requires the use of heavier clothing and equipment than most other endurance sports.

Clearly, if you have the proper skills and if you also have access to cross-country ski trails, this is an excellent choice for keeping your heart in shape. But those may be a couple of big "ifs," especially if you've never tried skiing or if you live in a warm climate.

Even if you are a good cross-country skier and live in the right geographical location, you will probably still find that you need an alternate endurance sport to pursue when the snow melts or when it's just not convenient to hit the trails. Running is an obvious warm-weather candidate, and I would certainly recommend it *if* the skier recognizes it's a different sport with different safety requirements. Dr. Stan James notes in an article in the February 1985 *Runner* that cross-country skiers incur most of their training injuries during summer running.

One great "summer supplement" for cross-country skiing is the "Nordic Track," which is a stationary device that can be used indoors to simulate skiing movements. This machine requires you to slide your feet and move your arms back and forth in the same way you do in actual cross-country skiing. Of course, you lose the added challenge of the cold air and heavy clothing and the thrill of being out of doors. But still, this device can provide a great aerobic workout. Although you may find that a good Nordic Track is a little too expensive to buy on your own, you might gain access to one in a gym or health club.

During the summer months in the Scandinavian countries, I've noticed that roller skiing is very popular. It's performed on a solid surface, using special ski poles and skis with rollers. This activity simulates cross-country skiing remarkably well, if it's done properly. I doubt if such exercise would ever be popular in this country, however, because of the lack of paved walking or bicycle paths, such as those found all over Europe and Scandinavia.

With either regular cross-country skiing, roller skiing, or the Nordic Track, you should work out for at least thirty minutes a day, a minimum of three and preferably four days a week, to achieve a good training effect.

Swimming

After cross-country skiing, swimming is the next best aerobic exercise, largely because it requires you to use many of the major muscles of your body. As with skiing, you should swim for twenty to thirty minutes at least four times a week to get adequate benefits for your cardiovascular system.

If you're a skillful swimmer, you can burn up quite a few calories in a short time. A swimmer will range from burning 5 calories to 20 calories a minute, depending on the speed and the stroke.

There are a number of advantages that swimming has over many of the other endurance activities. For example, it's much easier on your muscles and skeletal structure, mainly because of the natural buoyancy of the water. As a result, you'll be less likely to confront such things as knee and ankle problems and shin splints.

But it's not all sweetness and light in the pool. A person who lacks good technique, for instance, may find it impossible to go for the minimum twenty minutes without stopping several times to rest. Also, not every community has a pool available twelve months out of the year. Finally, at one time or another, most swimmers encounter infections of the eyes, ears, and nose. So, it's very important to choose effective items, such as nose plugs and goggles.

But even if you start out in relatively bad shape and with poor stroking ability, you may still find that swimming is just the sport for you. One dentist I know from Fort Worth, Texas, Dr. Wayne Peavey, started out a little slow, but he's roaring along now as a regular swimmer who is in tip-top shape.

About three years ago, when Wayne was approaching the disturbing age of forty, he decided he should do something about getting in shape. "I kept hearing about young men in their early forties having coronaries," he said. "So I decided I'd better get into some kind of exercise program to try to avoid future heart problems."

As a result, he began exercising in the gym room in the Downtown YMCA in Dallas. "I did a little light weight exercise, using things like the Nautilus," he recalled. "Then, I decided to try swimming. The first time I went to the pool, I was impressed by how some guys could swim back and forth, lap after lap without stopping. I thought, 'Goodness, they must be real he-men to be able to do that!' "

But as impressed as he was, Wayne wasn't intimidated—even

when he found that he couldn't make it from one end of the pool to the other without stopping. "I got completely winded!" he confessed. "In fact, I was so unsure of my swimming ability that I was afraid at first of going into the deep end of the pool because I thought I might drown. Actually, I realize now that even though I had been in the water before, I really didn't even know how to swim."

But Wayne kept at it. Gradually, by watching other people and picking up bits of information from instructors, he began to improve his stroke so that he finally developed a good crawl. From the outset, he has also observed some simple procedures that have kept him completely free of common swimming ailments. Unlike many new swimmers, he started out the right way by using ear plugs and goggles. As a result, he says he's never had any infections.

"I worked my way up from two laps in the pool to six or seven," he said. "Then, the distance increased steadily until now, I find myself swimming a little more than a mile. I feel that's probably enough for me—anything beyond that might border on fanaticism."

Wayne swims six days a week—every day except Sunday. It takes him about thirty-three minutes to swim his daily mile, and he also works out on the Nautilus three days a week. Now, it does take him some time to accomplish all this: He has to schedule two hours of each day for his exercise because of the need to travel back and forth to the pool, and also to shower and change clothes.

Even though Wayne's program has taken some time and commitment, it's really paid off in improved fitness. In 1981, just before he began his swimming program, he lasted only fifteen and three-quarters minutes on the treadmill stress test. That would have placed him in the "fair" category of fitness for males his age.

But then, after he embarked on his swimming program, his fitness began to soar. In 1983, he was able to do twenty-five minutes on the treadmill, and that put him up onto "superior" level. In his latest tests, his time was 27 minutes, three seconds—a performance that puts him in the ninety-ninth percentile of all those in his age group, regardless of how they exercise.

There are a couple of important lessons to learn from Wayne's experience. First of all, if you think you'd like to try swimming, don't let your lack of skill stop you. All you need is sufficient motivation and patience to stick with it until your technique improves.

Secondly, it's clear that a swimming program will put a person in top shape for the treadmill stress test—even though this test involves walking movements that are quite different from any swimming strokes. In other words, superior fitness will become clear on the treadmill stress test no matter what sport you pursue.

Jogging or Running

By the definition I use, jogging involves movement that's slower than nine minutes per mile, and running involves moving faster than nine minutes per mile. However you define it, running or jogging is perhaps the most popular aerobic exercise because it's the easiest and cheapest to do. Almost anyone can buy a pair of jogging shoes and shorts. Then, you just step outside and start putting one foot in front of the other.

But as easy as this sport may seem, I do want to offer a few words of caution for beginners. After all, the thing we're most concerned with in this book is safety, and for the jogger, that encompasses at least two levels: safety for your heart, and safety for your muscles, bones, and joints.

As for your heart, it's important to observe closely the four basic phases of sensible aerobic exercise outlined in the previous chapter. The cool-down is particularly important for reasons we've already discussed.

Generally speaking, I think the main guidelines for getting the maximum protection against heart disease and sudden death should start with this premise: *Begin slowly and never overdo it.*

Specifically, if you're running mainly for cardiovascular fitness, you should run for twenty to thirty minutes a session, four times a week. The maximum mileage I recommend is 12 to 15 miles a week. I've found from my own experience and studies that anything more isn't really necessary for achieving sufficient levels of fitness. And too much more—say the 60 or more miles a week Jim Fixx was running—could put you in great danger if you have any underlying heart problems.

As for avoiding injury to your muscles, bones, and joints, keep in mind these four "S's" and one "O":

• *Stretch.* Remember the warm-up routine we discussed in the last chapter.

• *Shoes.* Try on several pairs, and keep in mind the type of surface you'll be running on. The harder the surface, the more cushioning you need in your footwear.

• *Surface.* The surface on which you run has a direct effect on injuries. The worst surface is concrete; the best is one of the synthetic cushioned surfaces, like those found on many tracks. The next best surface would be a smooth, grassy field or a dirt road. A properly cared-for cinder track is also a good surface. Black-top or macadam is next to concrete as being one of the worse surfaces. If you have no choice but to exercise on a hard, nonresilient surface, that makes the selection of the proper shoe even more important.

Also, try to pick a course which is fairly flat. Although highly conditioned, competitive runners may use steep hills separately for intense training, very hilly terrain may place too much stress and strain on the average person's legs and ankles. It may also overload your cardiovascular system if you have underlying coronary problems.

Finally, it's important to be careful of traffic. A recent report from New Jersey indicated that one of the greatest causes of injuries among joggers there was automobile accidents.

• *Style.* Concentrate on keeping your entire body, including your neck and arms, as loose and free-moving as possible. Also, run with a rolling (or "pronating") heel-to-toe movement. And avoid trying to run distances primarily on your toes or the balls of your feet. Finally, avoid allowing your body to do any excessive bouncing because this places too much strain on your joints and bones.

• *Overuse.* Dr. Stan James, writing in the February 1985 issue of *The Runner,* says that training errors in running include "high mileage, high intensity and *sudden changes* in the program." Such practices lead to what I call "overuse" of the body and may result in ailments like musculo-skeletal problems, jogger's anemia, pseudonephritis of jogging (bleeding from the kidneys), and amenorrhea, or the cessation of menstruation.

Recent studies at the Institute for Aerobics Research in Dallas have shown that the injury level is minimal for those running 1 to 20 miles per week. But then the injuries increase exponentially from 20 to 40 and from 40 to 60 miles per week. So the solution to overuse ailments is to cut your mileage down. And again, I would emphasize the point I've frequently made before: If you run more than 15 miles per week, you're running for some reason other than cardiovascular fitness.

Also, it's interesting that each October at the Aerobics Center, when we recognize those people who run over 100 miles in the month, the running injuries skyrocket. The reason is that people who ordinarily run 12 to 15 miles a week quickly work up to 25 to 30 miles a week. But you can't just double your mileage in a short time and expect to avoid injuries. So if you plan to increase the amount of your exercise, be sure to do it gradually!

Some people love to run, but they want the option of doing it in the privacy of their own home. For these indoor athletes, an alternative to consider is the motorized treadmill. This device has a moving belt that can run at different speeds and also an incline adjustment that can give you the added demands of a gradual uphill run. There are also self-propelled treadmills which are sold in some shops, but I wouldn't recommend them. They are relatively difficult to use and ineffective in giving you the best workout.

For runners or joggers with recurrent injuries, I've found that exercising on a mini-trampoline has merit. Yet, the effect of gravity is neutralized to some extent on this device, and so longer periods of exercise are required than with running in place. Specifically, stationary running for twenty minutes, four times per week, can produce a training effect; in contrast, to get a training effect on a mini-trampoline requires thirty minutes, four times per week.

Outdoor Cycling

This sport, one of my "top five" for aerobic conditioning, builds strong leg muscles, and it's great for building cardiovascular endurance. Another advantage is that it's easier on your bones and joints than jogging.

Still, there are special hazards that the cyclist has to consider: You'll probably find that no matter where you exercise, you'll have to maneuver your bike in and out of some traffic, and that increases your risk of an accident. Also, the likelihood of falling off a bike or getting into an accident is increased by such factors as bad weather conditions, potholes on the road, and the possibility of a sudden distraction, such as a barking dog charging at your wheel.

Because of these traffic- and speed-related problems, it's essential that you buy a good crash helmet and wear it *every time* you take your bike out. The most serious cycling injuries involve the head. The material of the helmet should be strong enough so that it won't crack if you fall. This means you should consider something made of a very tough substance like aerospace plastic. The helmet should also be lined with foam for greater comfort, increased safety, and a better fit. A good helmet may cost from about $40 to $60.

As far as the bicycle itself is concerned, I'd recommend one of the three- to ten-speed varieties. A one-speed bike is too difficult for most people to pedal, especially on any sort of incline. On the other hand, considerably less energy is required using one of the multispeed bikes, and you must work harder to get a good training effect.

Before you go out for a spin on your bike, always check your tires, brakes, and gears. Too many accidents occur when a worn tire blows or faulty brakes fail to hold. If you're just starting a cycling program after being away from a bicycle for years, it's best to start out slowly to get the "feel" of the machine again. No matter how good you may have been as a youngster, you have to expect your reactions to be rusty at first after a long layoff.

As every cyclist knows, accidents can still happen even to highly conditioned and experienced cyclists. With the advent of triathlons, interest in cycling began to increase in the past few years, particularly among competitive runners. One of the outstanding marathoners at the Aerobics Center began training regularly for the local triathlons and obtained all the proper equipment for swimming and cycling. Nonetheless, while cycling at a high rate of speed downhill, he lost control of his bike, went over the handlebars, and struck his head.

Immediate medical attention didn't reveal any major injury, but persistent and severe pain prompted him to seek additional consultation. X-rays at the time showed several of the vertebrae in his neck were broken, and one was shattered! He could have become paralyzed from the neck down with any further movement, so surgery was performed on an emergency basis. Then, he had to wear a metal halo for almost three months. But he continued to walk to keep in shape aerobically.

His program turned out to be quite effective. The neck healed without complications, and less than five months following the accident, this man, who was in his early forties, ran a marathon in slightly over three hours, just a few minutes off his all-time record!

If you're a beginner, starting slowly on your program is safer and, physically, the wisest course for your heart. If you're out of shape, it will take several weeks for your muscles and endurance to build up. In fact, I would suggest that you give yourself at least ten weeks to work up to a 15 m.p.h. cruising speed. At this rate, you'll be doing a mile in four minutes, and that's fast enough. Anything faster is racing speed and not really necessary to achieve an adequate aerobic training effect. If you can cycle 5 miles in twenty minutes four or five times a week, you'll find you're involved in an effective and challenging training program.

Indoor Cycling

It's easier to achieve an aerobic training effect by cycling out of doors than it is if you work out on a stationary bike. The reason for this is that when you're on a real bicycle, you have the added burden of propelling your body weight forward. Also, you have to work against the resistance of the terrain and the wind. Still, a stationary bike, if it's used the right way, can do wonders for increasing your level of cardiovascular fitness.

One of the best illustrations I've encountered of what a stationary cycling routine can do for a highly motivated person involves Dr. Arnie Jensen, a 55-year-old radiologist at our Cooper Clinic. About eight years ago, he started an exercise program by jogging. But he found he couldn't run around the block without getting winded. And he ran into another problem. As his condition improved, he discovered he couldn't run enough to get a proper training effect because the exercise bothered his knee. He had an old football injury, and his knee started flaring up because of the jarring effect of his feet repeatedly hitting the pavement.

So he decided to try cycling on a stationary bike, and he quickly found that the pedaling didn't bother his knee at all. "As a matter of fact, my knee got better with the bike," he added.

Arnie embarked on a regular aerobic training program with a stationary bike, and before long, this out-of-shape radiologist had reached the "superior" level of fitness on our treadmill stress test at the Aerobics Center. In fact, in 1984, he set the Cooper Clinic record for the fifty-five to fifty-nine year age group with a time of 30:35!

How exactly did he do it? The first step was to get a good machine and put it where he was most likely to use it. Arnie has two bikes now, a Dynavit, which is a West German make, and a Schwinn Air-Dyne Ergometer. He keeps one in his office and uses the other one at home.

"The main thing is to get a bike with a 'flywheel,' which is a weighted wheel that makes the pedaling smooth," he says. "Or you might buy one like the Air-Dyne, where you can use your arms and legs together. With the Air-Dyne, you can condition both your arm and leg muscles—your arms go forward and backward as your legs go up and down. This way, you can do a higher level of endurance work without tiring out one set of muscles too quickly."

Arnie believes it's especially important for stationary bikers to get a machine that has a smooth action. "Some of the stationary bikes have the resistance clamped down on the pedals, without a flywheel, and that results in a jerky movement," he explains. "If your pedaling isn't smooth, your legs will give out too quickly."

The cost of a good stationary bike, by the way, will generally begin at about $600 and can go as high as $2,500 to $3,500. Those in the upper price ranges usually provide electronic computations for the resistance you're placing on the pedals. Also, they allow you to keep a record of the resistance you ride at daily and even monitor your heartbeat.

Arnie's exercise program consists of all the systematic, safe steps we've been discussing throughout this book. On the Air-Dyne, he begins with a basic three-minute warm-up. Then, he starts his aerobic phase. He pedals for about thirty-five to forty minutes at an effort level, marked on the machine, of 5–6; for the last two to three minutes, he'll increase his pedaling to a level of 7.

When Arnie works out on the Dynavit, he warms up at 120–200 watts, and then does twenty-five minutes of aerobic work at between 230 and 280 watts.

With both machines, he goes through a cool-down by pedaling on the bike with little or no resistance for about five minutes. Arnie follows these stationary cycling procedures four to five times a week. Also, he begins every day with 100 consecutive situps on an incline board and sixty push-ups on a push-up bar. It's obvious, isn't it, why he has managed to get into such superior physical condition!

Walking

Walking may seem as though it places too little demand on your body to qualify as an effective endurance exercise, but nothing could be further from the truth. As a matter of fact, walking ranks among the top five aerobic activities in the benefits it can produce in your body. As I said earlier, it just takes longer to achieve the same level of fitness with walking than with running or some of the more strenuous activities.

All it takes to be a walker is a good pair of comfortable, supportive walking shoes, with a sole thick enough to protect your feet from bruises. Any pair of good jogging shoes will serve the purpose quite well.

Walking is an outstanding activity for those who are susceptible to the joint, bone or muscle injuries that may accompany running. But as I say, you have to be able to put in some extra time if you want to be a walker. In other words, you should work up to walking about three miles in forty-five minutes. Also, it's necessary to follow this routine four to five times a week if you plan to use walking as your sole conditioner.

It's possible, however, to cut your exercise time and increase the benefits of walking by going uphill at the same pace that you move along a flat surface. Also, you might try carrying some Heavy Hands, the small weights we discussed in the previous chapter, to increase the demands on your body.

How well can a walking program condition your heart and improve your endurance level? The answer is *quite* well!

Our current record on the Balke treadmill stress test for walkers is twenty-seven minutes, established by a 57-year-old man. To achieve that performance, which is superior (or in the top 5 percent), even for men under thirty years of age, this man walks 5 miles, five days per week. His pace is quite rapid in that he averages twelve and one-half to thirteen minutes per mile. At that speed, he is exercising at about 65 percent of his maximal heart rate, and this accounts for his phenomenal level of fitness, as reflected by his treadmill performance.

Aerobic Dancing

As the benefits of endurance exercise become better known, new activities often appear on the horizon. Some are fly-by-night concepts that are here today and gone next year. But a few move beyond the fad stage to become staples of aerobic activity. One of these is aerobic dancing, which has become extremely popular and has shown considerable "staying power" on the exercise scene in recent years. It's estimated that in 1984, 18 million people, most of them women, were dancing for exercise.

Despite the possible aerobic benefits, however, recent surveys have revealed that there is a high injury rate that goes along with aerobic dancing. One study done by Dr. Douglas Richie, a podiatrist from Seal Beach, California, showed that 78 percent of the instructors and 43 percent of the students questioned had been injured while dancing. The most vulnerable area was the shins, followed by the feet, back, knees, calves, and hips.

Despite the potential dangers, however, it's not necessary to get hurt if you choose dancing. There are a number of simple ways to ascertain whether or not you're getting into a reputable program, and also to protect yourself against injury.

First of all, when you choose a dancing program, don't sign up for any classes until you've looked the facilities over, made some inquiries, and observed at least one class. It's also important to avoid shoestring operations that are more interested in packing their classes with paying customers than they are in providing a safe, effective service. I'd never pick a place that tried to high-pressure me into membership.

While you're looking the place over, you should ask about the surface on which you'll be dancing. The ideal floor is hardwood suspended on springs over an air space. Never dance on a floor that has no give to it—that's the way shin splints occur.

When you observe a class, notice if there is sufficient space for each student to move around, or if the class seems overcrowded. If the dancers are constantly bumping into one another's elbows and legs, you can bet that the incidence of injuries is higher than it should be. So ask about limits on class size.

It's important, too, to check the cleanliness of the place. If the floor on which you have to kneel and lie is filthy, that won't provide the most pleasant experience for a regular workout. Also, a complete aerobic dance facility may include equipment for weight-training and showers, and must be properly air-conditioned and heated.

Next, take a good look at the instructors. An instructor should be a trained professional who conducts the class with a warm-up period, an aerobic phase, and an adequate cool-down. The instructors should be in good shape themselves and should be sensitive to the needs of individual students. One way to check this is to see how often they watch and communicate with individual students. The best places will have the students monitor their heart rates periodically, particularly during recovery.

If proper, safe procedures haven't been instituted, or if a dance instructor isn't aware of how to respond to emergencies, students may find themselves in potentially dangerous situations. One terrified woman who came into our clinic recently had faced just such a situation.

She was almost forty-nine years old when she joined her aerobic dance class, and during one of her early exercise sessions, she had noticed that her heart rate would jump rapidly from 135 beats per minute to a rate in excess of 200 beats per minute.

When she mentioned this to the instructor, she was told, "Don't worry about that. Just go sit down for a while."

As we'll see, this wasn't very good advice, but she did sit down. And luckily, her heart rate eventually returned to normal. So she decided to continue in the dance program.

But then the same thing happened again. When she told her husband about what had been happening to her, he became alarmed. He insisted she come to our clinic for an evaluation, and we gave her a treadmill stress test. The test revealed that at a rate of 135 heartbeats per minute, her heart began to beat very rapidly in the pattern called ventricular tachycardia.

We stopped the stress test at this point, and almost immediately, the cardiac irregularity disappeared. But we knew we had to take further action. Due to the recurrent and possibly serious nature of her problem, we had her hospitalized for a diagnostic workup. It took five days to find the proper combination of medicines that could control this potentially fatal problem. If she had continued with those aerobic dance classes—and especially with the "sit-down-for-a-while" approach that had been prescribed—she might have suffered a fatal heart seizure.

There are also other safety measures you should check for when you're selecting an aerobic dance class. For example, you'll want to find out whether or not the program provides cardio-pulmonary resuscitation, in case someone has a heart problem. In my opinion, the presence of someone with CPR training is absolutely essential.

Finally, a good aerobics dance program will offer separate classes for beginning, intermediate, and advanced students. You wouldn't start out running at an eight-minute per mile pace if you were a jogger; by the same token, you wouldn't want to dance at an advanced level on your first day in one of these classes.

A dance program should be designed so that your capacity will increase gradually, until you're able to sustain your aerobic dance phase for twenty minutes without stopping. When you reach the point where you can do this three or four times a week, you'll find you're getting enough exercise for an aerobic training effect. In fact, you may find that the results are nothing short of amazing.

Take Diane Cadenhead, for example. She was a distance runner for many years, and at one time she ran regularly with my wife, Millie. Yet, after she passed forty years of age, she began to have chronic musculo-skeletal problems, primarily in her back. These difficulties eventually caused her to stop jogging, and as a substitute, she embarked on a progressive walking program.

But then, a move from Dallas to Minneapolis prompted her to change her program again because the long winters made year-round walking outdoors too unpleasant. Finally, Diane enrolled in an aerobic dancing program, and she worked up to one hour of activity, three to four times per week. On some days, time permitting, she would complete two classes for a total of two hours.

I've been following Diane regularly over the past thirteen years, and as long as she was running, her best Balke treadmill performance was twenty minutes. But after two years into her aerobic dancing program we tested her again, and this time, she added four minutes to her all-time record. This twenty-four minute performance placed her in the superior category of fitness for women under thirty years of age—and she was forty-nine.

So clearly, aerobic dancing, if done properly, can be very effective in improving cardiovascular fitness. But still, a few cautionary words are in order about this activity. I mentioned four "S's" and an

"O" when we discussed the safe approach to running, and you'll find that they apply to dancing as well.

• *Stretch.* A warm-up, with plenty of stretching exercises, is especially important for a dancer because of the stresses and strains that are put on the muscles and joints.

• *Shoes.* There are some specially designed shoes that can help aerobic dancers avoid injury. More flexible than running shoes, they have a cushioned inner sole made of durable, spongy material that absorbs the impact of jumping. The heel cup should be solid and stiff, and the sole of the shoe should flare slightly at the heel to provide stability. There are no outstanding shoes at this time, though some are designed strictly for aerobic dancing. These are better than standard running or jogging shoes, which should be avoided.

• *Surface.* As I've said, suspended wood floors are the best. If you have no choice but to use hard floors, try covering them with a plastic-covered foam mat.

• *Style.* Dance lightly and try to glide, rather than bounce vigorously.

• *Overuse.* If you do three to four hours of dancing per week (e.g., in four forty–five minute sessions), you'll be in a safe range. But if you begin to do more than five hours a week, you'll be more likely to suffer one or more of those injuries we discussed earlier.

Above all, don't try to achieve what some aerobic programs have called the "burn." If you feel a burning sensation in your chest or trunk, that could be a heart or coronary problem, which is certainly the kind of thing you want to avoid. If any of your other muscles feel as though they are burning, they are probably signalling to you that they're overworked and perhaps on the verge of injury.

This discussion of the merits and safety features of various aerobic activities could go on indefinitely. But I think that by now you can see the major principles of safety and soundness to keep in mind for most sports. The main idea is to choose an exercise program that will get your heart rate up to your "target" level. At the same time, the program should involve a minimum of risk both to your muscles, bones, and joints on the one hand, and to your heart on the other.

But to find an approach that will provide maximum protection for your heart, something else is required. You can be as cautious as you like in selecting a program and still be in danger unless you move beyond the "do-it-yourself" approach to exercise. That means checking out the precise condition of your heart through a properly conducted treadmill stress test—the procedure I regard as the master key to good health and exercising without fear.

CHAPTER SEVEN

THE STRESS TEST: THE KEY TO GOOD HEALTH AND A LONGER LIFE

Suppose I told you that tomorrow you could take a single, safe test which is able to:

- determine with great reliability whether you are currently suffering from coronary heart disease;
- indicate the likelihood you have for developing coronary artery disease in the future;
- tell you exactly the present level of your cardiovascular fitness; and
- help your doctor prescribe a safe and effective exercise program.

You might think that I was making outlandish claims for a test that simply doesn't exist. And if it does, the cost for taking such a test must be prohibitively expensive.

Fortunately, these claims are true, and the test is not excessively expensive. In fact, I've been using such a test at the Aerobics Center in Dallas for years. Physicians all over the world have found this testing to be of great value in their practice of medicine.

What I'm referring to is the treadmill stress test, which in recent years has been fine-tuned to such a degree that today it can often tell you much of what you might want to know about the state of your heart and cardiovascular system.

Although we've mentioned this concept in prior pages, you may still wonder exactly what I mean by stress testing. Generally speaking, the test measures the performance of the heart while it is working hard, such as during exercise.

To make accurate comparisons among patients, the exercise and test procedure have been carefully standardized. In this way, doctors and technicians can measure such things as blood pressure, heart rate, and oxygen use. Most important of all, they monitor the electrical impulses of the heart by taking an electrocardiogram. Because a proper stress test involves a standard routine, your body's reactions can be evaluated against the performance of other people. That way, we can tell whether you're "normal" or not.

The type of exercise you may be asked to do during a stress test can vary from clinic to clinic. In some cases, stationary exercise bicycles are used; in others, treadmills are standard. Some clinics avoid equipment altogether. Instead, the doctors instruct their patients to walk over some steps or just run in place.

Whatever approach is employed, the testing procedure should encourage the patient to attain his "maximum heart rate," so that the heart is operating at close to peak capacity. As we've seen in a previous chapter, to find your predicted maximum heart rate (PMHR), we use the following formula: For men, it is 205 minus one-half the person's age. For women, it's 220 minus the age. So, a 40-year-old man has a PMHR of 185 beats per minute. A 40-year-old woman has a PMHR of 180. In the testing laboratory, we use age-adjusted and fitness-adjusted predicted maximum heart rates, as shown in the chart in the Appendix.

Testing at this maximal capacity gives a more accurate picture of the condition of the heart. Among other things, it's much more likely to reveal heart disorders that may not surface at rest or at less rigorous levels of exercise testing. In fact, "submaximal" testing, or testing which involves only 85 percent of a person's maximum heart rate, may miss as many as 39 percent of heart disorders that would be revealed by maximal testing.

As I see it, there are at least five important reasons a stress test can be of value to you:

Reason #1:   To Provide Motivation to Exercise

A periodic stress test can be a wonderful motivational tool. Once you see where you stand in relation to the thousands of other people who have taken the test, you will get a much more realistic view of what you need to do to improve your level of fitness. You'll also understand more fully the ways you can enhance your protection against heart disease and sudden death.

By comparing the results of one of your tests to the next, you can also measure personal improvement in your level of fitness. In this way, the stress test can reinforce the personal exercise program you've chosen by showing your precise rate of progress. The test has been refined so much that it can measure improvement or deterioration in your fitness even when you yourself may not notice any difference.

Also, on the basis of the results of your stress test, you may choose to alter your exercise routine in a way that can be more beneficial. One man who is a regular at our Aerobics Center was running two fairly fast miles a day, four days a week, and he scored precisely at the beginning of the superior level for his age group. But he wasn't satisfied.

Although his level of cardiovascular fitness was outstanding, he said he sometimes felt a little sluggish and lacked energy at the end of the day.

So I recommended that he change his program. Specifically, he increased his running to 2.5 miles a day but at a slightly slower pace, four days a week. I told him if he followed this routine, he would probably see an improvement in his test time.

Apparently, this was enough to motivate him for a full year to change his approach to working out. The next year when he came in for his treadmill stress test, his time, still in the top superior category, had gone up by one-and-a-half minutes! Moreover, he felt better and reported that his level of energy had improved.

A regular stress test, if it's done with the latest techniques and procedures, can be a wonderful tool for motivation. It can show you graphically, in black and white, whether your exercise program is doing you any good, and also can help you decide whether or not you need to adjust your approach to conditioning.

Reason #2: To Provide Your Physician with Information on Your Level of Fitness

The test can give your physician a more precise idea of what level of exercise you can tolerate. For example, if you turn in a "poor" performance on the treadmill, no sensible doctor would tell you to try to run a complete twenty to thirty minutes the first time you embark on an exercise program. Rather, he'll be more likely to suggest that you walk the distance or, at the most, combine walking with some light jogging.

Also, if you are just starting to exercise after recovering from a heart attack, you must be aware of the limitations of your condition. If you exercise too strenuously, you may be placing yourself at risk. A treadmill stress test can show your physician exactly what's happening with your heart as your heart rate increases during exercise, from which he can give you an exercise prescription.

Reason #3: To Provide a Baseline for Future Reference

Having either a resting or a stress electrocardiogram as a baseline for future reference is immensely important. In fact, all patients coming to our Cooper Clinic now receive a credit-card-sized emergency card to keep in their billfolds. On one side there is emergency data, and on the other side a copy of their resting ECG. On more than one occasion, physicians have told me how valuable that card was in helping to make a diagnosis.

Even though our patients don't carry a copy of their stress ECG with them, having one on file for comparative purposes is very important. If a test is normal year after year, and then it abruptly becomes abnormal (this is also referred to as a "serial change"), we can predict with great reliability that something abnormal has happened to the

heart. Our accuracy in detecting obstructive coronary disease rises
rapidly in such cases.

Reason #4:   To Help Determine Whether You Have Heart Disease

This is probably the most important use of the stress test. It is
also one of the most disputed. But the bulk of the evidence over the
past few years shows that when the test is properly administered and
interpreted, it can provide valuable information to a doctor when he
assesses a person's overall coronary risk.

Let's look at just how the test can help detect disease. As I mentioned earlier, the stress test monitors your body's response to exercise. As a matter of fact, just the length of time you can last on the
treadmill can tell a great deal about your health, even if sophisticated
heart-monitoring devices are not used.

In a recent scientific journal, Dr. R. M. Mills, Jr. and Dr. J. M.
Greenberg of the University of Massachusetts noted that patients
who perform well on the exercise aspect of the test have a far better
long-term chance of avoiding a heart attack or sudden death. They
went on to say that, even among patients who were known to have
coronary artery disease, the ability to achieve a heart rate of 160
beats per minute placed them in a low coronary risk group.

On the other hand, the researchers say, some patients taking a
treadmill stress test are at a much higher risk of heart attack and
sudden death. This group includes those people:

- who are unable to get their heartbeat above 120 beats per minute;
- who feel chest pain during exercise; or
- whose blood pressure falls during exercise.

Other studies have also shown that patients who were unable to
run for six minutes on one particular treadmill test had a higher rate
of coronary events over the next few years. The same is true for those
who experience pain during their peak exertion. In another study,
patients who had abnormal electrocardiograms or who quit very early
on in the treadmill test, had a poor rate of survival. Only 63 percent
were alive four years later.

Reason #5: To Predict Survival or Additional Heart Problems Following a Heart Attack

In recent years, the use of a submaximal stress test prior to discharge from the hospital following a documented heart attack has gained popularity. If the submaximal stress ECG is normal, the possibility of a severe problem within one year is minimal. To the contrary, an abnormal ECG at that time means the prognosis is guarded and more definitive measures might be indicated, including coronary artery bypass surgery.

So the exercise portion of the stress test *alone* gives important information about a patient's long-term prospects, even without considering other diagnostic tests.

Of course, I don't mean to downplay the importance of other measurements, and especially the electrocardiogram. As a matter of fact, the electrocardiogram is probably the most pivotal diagnostic tool associated with the stress test.

Here's the way it works: To get an effective electrocardiogram, discs called electrodes are placed at various points on the chest and, sometimes, on the back. Each of these electrodes helps to monitor the electrical impulses that occur with the contractions of the heart. Chapter 8 contains illustrations of this procedure.

Measurements of these impulses on an electrocardiogram can show if the flow of blood to a part of the heart is impeded or blocked. The doctor may conclude from such results that you should alter your diet or exercise program. Or perhaps you should go in for an arteriogram, so that the doctor can get a precise visual picture of the extent to which your arteries are clogged.

To take an electrocardiogram, the doctor attaches electrodes on your body to a series of wires, which in turn are hooked up to the electrocardiograph. This is an instrument that records the electrical impulses emitted by your heart as a series of sharply lined patterns on a graph.

With several electrodes, technicians can monitor the functioning of the heart from a variety of different directions, or "leads." Generally speaking, the greater the number of leads the clinician monitors, the more reliable or specific your ECG will be. If some part of your heartbeat is unusual or irregular, the lines on the electrocardiogram will most likely show this abnormality.

When an electrocardiogram is being taken, the electrical impulses from the heart are recorded automatically by a marker on a continuously moving roll of graph paper. In this way, each heartbeat creates a line, or "wave," with a series of spikes, or jagged up-and-down marks. Typically, each complete heartbeat contains a large, sudden upward spike, accompanied by smaller lines.

As you can see in Figure 1, each turning point of the line is labeled with a letter. A complete heartbeat, for instance, starts at an initial turning point—labeled with the letter "P." As the heart contraction continues, each turning point of the jagged line is labeled consecutively as points Q, R, S, and T. At T, the heart pauses momentarily—as indicated by a straight line on the electrocardiogram—before starting another heartbeat cycle, beginning with a new P.

The main thing you should focus your attention on is the last line on the electrocardiogram, before the electrical cycle ends and the

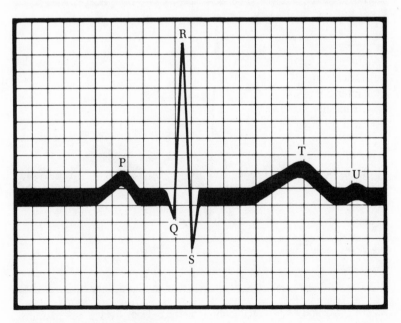

Figure 1. Normal ECG Tracing

pause, marked by the straight line, begins. Of course, the entire heart-beat cycle will be examined by your physician. But that last line of each contraction, which runs between points S and T, is considered to be of major importance in revealing heart disease. This key line, by the way, is known technically as the "S-T segment"—and it's often referred to this way in popular medical news reports. Figure 2 shows the S-T segment.

When the heartbeats are normal, the S-T segment follows a "normal" sharp incline. But at other times, this S-T segment may slope gently upward. In still other cases, the S-T line may not incline at all during the final phase of the heartbeat: Instead, it may decline, or form a horizontal "plateau." (See Figure 3.) These unusual movements may not be cause for great alarm, but they are reason to do further tests to evaluate the condition of the heart and arteries.

The course and shape of a normal S-T segment is relatively predictable from one human being to the next. In other words, people

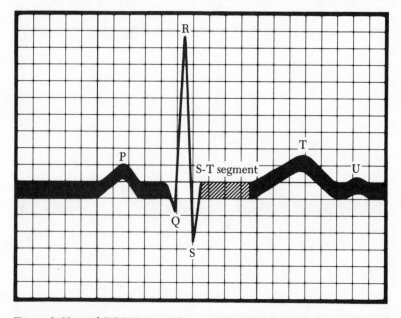

Figure 2. Normal ECG Tracing Showing the S-T Segment

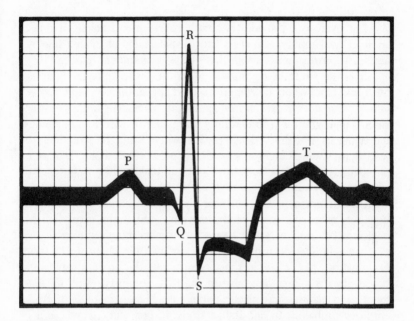

Figure 3. ECG Tracing Showing a Depressed S-T Segment

with healthy hearts and coronary arteries can expect their S-T segments to shoot directly upward before the next heart contraction
begins. On the other hand, when the S-T segment is irregular, or
"displaced" from its expected position, that's sometimes an indication of an abnormality in the flow of blood. The heart and coronary
arteries are giving an electrical "S.O.S." signal that the electrocardiogram is picking up. Often, when the doctor compares the abnormal
electrocardiogram with such things as heart rate, blood pressure, and
the length of time a person can exercise, an ECG abnormality becomes a reliable indicator of coronary disease.

After you take a treadmill stress test, your performance and other
health characteristics will be matched against your previous exams
and against those of other patients who have taken the identical test.
By comparing your results with the health histories of other people, a
doctor can make some determination about your relative health and
fitness, as well as your likelihood of having heart disease.

But even as I provide this crash course in cardiology, I don't want to oversimplify. Not every little displacement of the S-T line on an electrocardiogram is a sign that you're in imminent danger.

Suppose, for instance, that the S-T line is less than one millimeter off course from where it ordinarily should appear on the graph. Either you or your doctor can clearly see this displacement because every electrocardiogram is recorded on graph paper divided into one-millimeter blocks. But this little aberration, while it may be something to watch, isn't something you should get too worried about. That is, a one-millimeter displacement may not be all that significant. Often, we refer to such readings as "equivocal."

An S-T segment that is more than one millimeter off course, however, is usually considered abnormal. And if the displacement measures two millimeters or more, that is even more significant.

Now, in specific terms, if these irregularities show up in your examination, just what do they mean about the condition of your heart? Since 1962, studies have shown that certain types of S-T segment abnormalities may place a patient at a higher risk of death from coronary problems. In one Italian study, in fact, patients whose S-T segments went off course by one millimeter or more during exercise had 5.5 times greater risk of coronary events over the next few years.

Recently, there has been some criticism of the use of stress testing on the grounds that it's not accurate enough to predict the presence or risk of heart disease. So, just how reliable are these tests?

The criticisms have generally focussed on those tests which aren't conducted properly. Clearly, if the test uses only three chest electrodes, a great deal of what's going on in the heart during exercise is going to be missed. Also, if the approach fails to bring the person being tested up to a maximum heart rate during the test, other possible problems with the heart and coronary arteries may slip through undetected.

To avoid mistakes, we use fourteen electrodes, a technique which monitors fifteen "leads" of the heart, at the Aerobics Center. We also test all our people at their maximum heart rates. With these and other safeguards, which we'll discuss in more detail in the next chapter, we've found that we can minimize the large majority of false readings and mistakes in the stress test.

In short, I have become convinced after twenty-four years of experience that those treadmill stress tests which are properly conducted can be remarkably accurate. And others who follow sophisticated testing procedures have come to the same conclusion.

In one recent study, Dr. Peter Stone of the Harvard Medical School reported that of the patients whose S-T segments were irregular by more than 2.5 millimeters, *none* had healthy heart vessels. In fact, about 90 percent with S-T displacement this far off course turned out to have disease in several coronary vessels.

Furthermore, if your S-T segment continues to be abnormal even *after* exercise, that, too, can be a strong indicator of disease. According to Dr. Stone, more than 40 percent of patients whose ECG returned to normal within a minute of exercise had normal arteries or single vessel disease. But in patients whose S-T segments continued to be abnormal for at least nine minutes after a workout, 90 percent were shown to have multivessel disease.

So, the value of the stress test is obvious: A doctor who conducts the test properly and detects and confirms any irregularities early will be in a position to recommend treatment that could save your life.

Still, I don't want to be a Pollyanna about this. The ECG taken during maximum exercise isn't perfect. Even significant irregularities don't automatically mean that you definitely have heart disease. There are many other risk factors that a doctor must consider before ordering further tests. When the evidence strongly points to a high risk of heart disease, a doctor must rely on his best judgment about whether or not to get more "conclusive" testing.

To determine whether further tests should be conducted, the doctor, among other things, will examine the results of your stress test in even more depth. He knows it's not just the amount of displacement of the S-T line that is important. He will also look at *the time* during the exercise test when this abnormality occurs.

For example, it's more serious if the S-T displacement occurs while the patient is at rest, or if it appears early in a stress test at "sub-maximal" exercise levels. In such a case, it's much more likely that some heart disease is present. If abnormalities occur at these points, the odds are that the patient is a prime candidate for this more "conclusive" testing.

Now, what exactly is this conclusive testing? If better tests exist, you may well wonder, why not just give them to everybody in the first place?

Unfortunately, it's not as easy as all that, because the more accurate tests carry higher risks to the patient. For example, if a doctor seriously suspects you have heart disease, he may suggest that you have a test called a coronary arteriogram. In this procedure, a thin tube (catheter) is inserted into an artery in the groin and then pushed up through the blood vessels into the heart. (See Figure 4.) During this examination, the arteries are filled with a substance that will show up on X-rays so that the physician can make a conclusive determination about whether arteriosclerosis is present.

But as I said, this test is not without some risk. Less than 1 percent suffer side effects as a result of this examination. The risk of serious complications or death is less than one-tenth of a percent in competent examiners. But still, an arteriogram is not something to be taken lightly, and a physician should only recommend it if he has strong suspicions of disease.

So, the much safer stress test is often the best first step to take. If that reveals a serious problem, your doctor may then recommend a coronary arteriogram. The arteriogram, in turn, will provide conclusive evidence for or against the existence of clogged arteries.

Since 1973, many patients, mostly without any symptoms, have come to the Cooper Clinic and have had a very abnormal stress test. From that group, we studied one hundred who were advised to have a coronary arteriogram. From the arteriogram, seventy-eight were shown to have serious disease. Out of that group of seventy-eight, forty-seven had coronary artery bypass surgery, and three had "balloon angioplasty" (where a balloon is expanded within the coronary artery to open it up by compressing the cholesterol deposits or plaques). The remainder of the patients followed "conservative" treatment by being placed in lifestyle-changing programs, such as low-fat diets and increased exercise.

Even though some of these patients have been followed for as long as eleven years, only two out of the total group of one hundred have died. In contrast, 5 to 10 percent of patients with severe coronary disease, as seventy-eight of the one hundred were shown to have, are expected to die each year. This illustrates dramatically the diagnostic value of early detection and treatment. Without some type of intervention, at least twenty of the seventy-eight should already have expired.

Despite the overwhelming evidence of the value of the stress test, however, some of my colleagues still heatedly dispute the value of exercise testing. For one thing, there are doctors who argue that stress

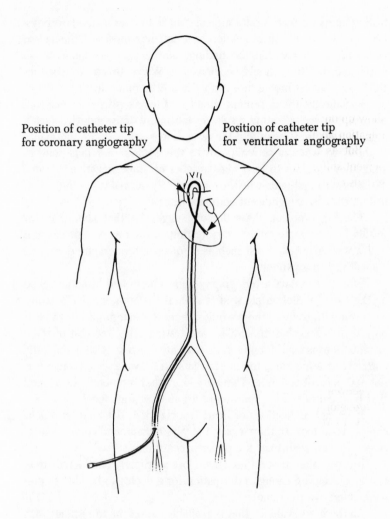

Position of catheter tip
for coronary angiography

Position of catheter tip
for ventricular angiography

Figure 4. Cardiac Catheterization

testing offers no more useful information than does a standard physical combined with an evaluation of a patient's history. Others even go so far as to say that the findings of the tests are generally so unreliable that they should be dismissed. We've already touched on this topic, but let me go into it now in a little more detail.

Specifically, the dissenters often base their skepticism on the contention that stress testing results in too many "false positive" readings. By this, they mean that the tests show some sort of abnormality in the heart when none really exists. Also, some researchers point to what they consider to be a high number of "false negative" results. These occur in patients who show a perfectly normal stress test, when in fact they have significant coronary disease.

The big problem, these doctors suggest, is that abnormal test results may promote unnecessary testing, as well as patient concern and worry. After all, a test such as coronary arteriography does pose a small risk to a patient.

Prior to coronary arteriography, most clinics and hospitals relied on the use of radioisotopic studies such as thallium or MUGA scans. Yet even with some of these studies, there is a margin of error that is only slightly less than treadmill stress testing. Also, the cost of these examinations is considerably more than a stress test. At this time, the coronary arteriogram is the most reliable test available, although it is not 100 percent accurate. There are also other tests being developed that hold considerable promise but are not yet functional.

If enough indications of heart trouble exist, delaying treatment can be hazardous. In those cases, I always recommend coronary arteriography and then treat the patient accordingly.

But still, the question remains: Does a properly conducted stress test give accurate enough information for a doctor to be able to prescribe effective treatment?

All the hard evidence that is available causes me to respond with a resounding "Yes!" Now, let me show you, step by step, why I arrive at this enthusiastic conclusion.

The first fact you should be aware of is that there are very few stress tests that require a doctor to make a "judgment call" about further testing. Of 43,000 ECG stress tests given to men at the Cooper Clinic, we found that only 7.4 percent were clearly abnormal, and 6.5 percent were equivocal. In other words, about 86 percent were normal. Out of 8400 women tested, only 3.8 percent were abnormal, with 8.1 percent equivocal. Again, fully 88 percent were normal.

So now, let's assume we have a small group of positive stress tests. The question next becomes, "Are they false or true positives?" That is, are they signalling correctly that there is some sort of underlying heart disease, or are the signals we're getting simply inaccurate?

The criticism of stress testing has centered on the observation that only about 60 percent of the positive readings that emerge from a test turn out to be accurate. That is, coronary heart disease is really present.

But the other side of the story is that treadmill stress tests which follow more stringent procedures may be more than 80 percent on the mark. At the Aerobics Center, we regularly find that our positive readings are over 80 percent accurate when compared to coronary arteriography. Any diagnostic study used in the practice of medicine that has an 80 percent accuracy is felt to be of clinical value. Moreover, there are practically no tests used in medicine that are 100 percent accurate.

But now, what about the people with false *negatives*, or a test which reveals no abnormalities, even though there is some coronary problem?

The bad news is that we miss these people entirely with the stress test. The good news is that there are so few false negatives in our testing that the number is negligible. And those people we do miss are certainly no worse off than they were before taking the test. Their only problem is that because the test doesn't identify them at all, they may go away with a false sense of security.

Of course, I'm all in favor of minimizing the number of false readings on stress tests. So, it's crucial that the treadmill stress test be properly administered and interpreted. As I've indicated, many of the false readings can be avoided by refining the testing procedure. So, testing with just a few leads tends to result in more false readings than with multiple leads. Doctors should also note those patients who are taking drugs for hypertension or heart problems, because such medications can result in a false positive reading.

There are still other factors that reduce the reliability of many stress tests:

• Testing at submaximal levels—or those significantly below a person's maximum heart rate during exercise—is far less reliable than stress tests at maximal levels. Most physicians will test to only 85 percent of the predicted maximal heart rate because of the mistaken belief that this level of testing is safe and accurate. But as we mentioned before, 39 percent or more of the abnormals will be missed if you stop at 85 percent maximum.

From a more personal perspective, in light of my own experience, I have trouble understanding how anyone can say that maximal stress testing is dangerous. After all, I've been involved with more than 70,000 maximal performance tests over the past twenty-four years—and I've never had a death with stress testing! Clearly, with proper selection and monitoring of the patients, maximal stress testing can be safe and sensitive.

• Tests using exercise bicycles or repeated "stair-stepping" are not as reliable as those tests using treadmills.

Maximal bicycle performance is usually limited by leg weakness, except with trained cyclists. Far too often, a test has to be stopped with a low maximal heart rate because the person's legs "played out." With treadmill testing, however, maximal heart rates are easier to achieve.

• The Masters two-step test is less frequently used because maximal performance isn't reached and monitoring is limited to the pre- and post-exercise periods only. No monitoring is done during the actual test when considerable abnormality may be occurring.

• Finally, in some patients it's almost impossible to obtain an ECG tracing that can be interpreted accurately. For some reason, there is a wandering of the baseline tracing, both at rest and during exercise. Or there may be considerable inconsistency during the test. In these cases, we call the results "inconclusive."

Being aware of these factors and correcting for them should help a doctor interpret his findings more accurately.

I recognize, of course, that a stress test alone will not give a doctor conclusive proof of the presence or absence of coronary disease. Such things as patient history, family history of heart disease, blood profile, and other risk factors are also extremely important. But having said this, I still agree with a large body of researchers who believe that an abnormal exercise stress test should be considered an independent coronary risk factor.

Now, let's move on to some of the finer points of stress testing, so that you can get the most out of this master key to a healthy heart.

First of all, one test is not enough. For example, more serious testing, such as the coronary arteriogram, should rarely be recommended on the basis of the results of just one stress test and nothing else. In fact, I don't routinely recommend arteriograms even when some other risk factors are present with an abnormal exercise ECG. Instead, I prefer to be more conservative. When I look at a patient's stress test results, I first like to compare them with previous examples from the same patient. Studies have shown that the results of this kind of "serial testing" are far more likely to be reliable.

One of the reasons for regular testing is that slightly abnormal readings may occur consistently in an individual from year to year. But as long as the signals from the heart stay the same, there may be no cause for alarm. In fact, if there is no worsening on the ECG for many years and the person's other risk factors stay about the same, there may be no need for more serious tests.

One patient whom I worked with for fourteen years consistently had both an abnormal stress test and low-grade angina pains. But his condition has stayed stable, and his stress test didn't show progressive changes until January 1984.

At that time, when I told this man that his ECG had changed considerably for the worse, he said, "I'm not surprised to hear that. My chest pain has increased, too."

With that information, I ordered his first coronary arteriogram, which showed grossly abnormal clogging of the coronary arteries. Within a few days, he underwent quadruple coronary-artery bypass surgery. The operation went well, and a few weeks later he was back on his exercise program. A repeat stress test was normal.

Such cases show how the test can be used to make a decision about the necessity of conducting more extensive studies and procedures, including possible surgery. When a patient shows significant changes in his exercise ECG from one stress test to the next, he may well be in imminent danger. In such a case, swift action is required. That's why I recommend that people over the age of forty have an *annual* stress test to supply their doctor with the most up-to-date information.

To illustrate how effective stress testing can work in special situations, here are some cases of people with quite different personal health backgrounds. It's likely that you'll see things in their stories that remind you of yourself or of some loved one. So as you read, remember: Their lives were probably saved by regular stress tests— and yours may well be, too.

The Engineer with a Sudden Change of Heart

Harry, an engineer, started visiting our Clinic when he was fifty-seven years old. For many years, he was totally without symptoms— no chest pains or other discomfort. Also, he had what we call a rather "moderate" risk profile: no family history of coronary heart disease; no smoking habits; only moderate tension in his life; moderate body fat; and borderline hypertension.

His blood profile was also average, showing relatively moderate levels of cholesterol and triglycerides. Finally, on his first stress test in 1971, he was in the "fair" category, and he improved to the "excellent" level a few years later.

I would have liked for him to get in even better shape and improve his diet so that perhaps he might have moved into the "low" risk category. All in all, there was certainly nothing to be alarmed about—at least not on the surface. A doctor performing a standard physical would have thought Harry was just fine.

In fact, Harry continued to seem fine for quite some time. When we gave him his first treadmill stress test in 1971, he was normal, though there was an indication that he may have had a heart attack sometime in the past. As a result, we decided to watch him fairly closely. For several years afterward, however, it seemed our concern might have been unwarranted because he continued to have normal test results. But then some troubling signs started to crop up.

By 1978, seven years after he first started coming in, Harry complained of some mild chest pain during exercise. Also, during the maximal phase of the treadmill workout when his heart was working hardest, his electrocardiogram showed some distressing "notching" that had never appeared before.

"Harry," I told him, "it looks like we're going to have to classify your stress test as 'abnormal' this time."

"Is it really bad?" he asked.

"Not yet, but if it gets any worse, we're going to be concerned. Are you getting much exercise?"

"Oh, I take a brisk walk once or twice a week, and I play a round of golf now and then."

"Well, you better do more than that," I told him. "Lose some weight, and try to be more active."

But I guess I wasn't too persuasive. Contrary to my advice, he stopped nearly all of his exercise. It's quite possible that by cutting back on exercise, he accelerated his disease. In the next couple of years, his condition continued to gradually decline.

Finally, by 1982, we followed up with yet another stress test. Before the test, his resting ECG showed some irregularities, but they were very slight. Our best guess at this stage was to classify the readings as "probably normal." That's as far as most physicians who don't use stress testing would have gone, and Harry would probably have walked out of the exam with a conviction that all was right in his world.

We took things a step further. We put him on the treadmill for a maximal performance stress test, and as it turned out, this was the best thing that could have happened to him. Before long, some clear danger signals began to show up.

For one thing, his maximum heart rate stayed unusually low: It never exceeded 140 beats per minute. A person his age—he was in his early sixties—should have been able to attain at least 160 beats per minute. Finally, at fifteen minutes into the treadmill test, he developed some chest pain, though he kept running for two more minutes before quitting.

Most important of all, Harry's stress ECG was much worse than it had been on his previous test. When we saw this clear deterioration, we decided that Harry was now in serious danger. So we put him in the hospital for a coronary arteriogram. As we had suspected, his coronary arteries were severely clogged with arteriosclerosis. In fact, he required triple bypass surgery.

The combination of stress test, arteriogram, and bypass surgery may well have saved his life. As I've said, a routine physical wouldn't have detected his disease. As a result, he might have become another victim of sudden death. Instead, he recovered completely from his surgery, and on his most recent treadmill stress test, he lasted for more than nineteen minutes, a performance which put him well up into the excellent category of fitness.

Of course, not everybody's condition declines as gradually as did Harry's. In some people, the changes that occur happen so fast that each day that goes by without treatment can add significantly to the risk. That's why, as you'll see in the next example, I think people over forty should have a stress test once a year.

The Banker Who Can Now Count on a Longer Life

When Gene, a fiftyish banker from West Texas, came into the Aerobics Center, he liked to "keep tabs on the old ticker," as he put it, with a regular stress test. And for ten years Gene's results were consistently normal. He certainly seemed to be in pretty good overall shape, and if a doctor had given Gene a routine physical, the prognosis would probably have been that Gene was the picture of health.

But the doctor would have been wrong—dead wrong.

You see, something suddenly happened that a routine physical wouldn't have picked up. But because Gene was in the habit of having a regular stress test, we noticed an alarming development: For the first time ever, his stress ECG became grossly abnormal.

Of course, a person can have an abnormal ECG and still not be in imminent danger of a coronary event. But when we see a sudden worsening of an ECG from one test to the next, or a steady build-up of other risk factors, we generally consider that a sign of trouble. With a minor abnormality on the ECG, we can often assume that the danger is slight. But Gene's electrocardiogram showed such a strong irregularity that I felt it just couldn't be ignored.

I sent Gene for a thallium scan, a test in which radioisotopic material is inserted into the heart and then scanned with a special instrument that will often show disease that is present. The test came back negative, however, indicating there was apparently no disease. Gene breathed a sigh of relief, naturally thinking that the electrocardiograph was just "on the blink."

But I wasn't convinced.

First of all, I have a lot of faith in the stress tests we conduct at the Clinic. I know they're not perfect, but usually they are highly reliable predictors of heart disease. This time, the change in the ECG had seemed to be too clear-cut to dismiss.

Secondly, I knew the thallium scan itself was not a foolproof test. After further discussions, I finally convinced the banker to have a coronary arteriogram, which would be a far more conclusive test.

Sure enough, the arteriogram showed significant coronary artery disease. As a result, Gene underwent a life-saving bypass operation.

So in this case, a treadmill stress test picked up heart disease where a routine physical and a thallium scan failed. And Gene picked up a few more years to "watch his ticker."

A major point in this story is the fact that Gene had undergone *regular* stress tests. This meant we were able to catch his disease just as it took a turn for the worse; if the condition had gone undetected for a longer period, he might have found himself in big trouble.

Unfortunately, many people haven't followed the lead of wise patients like Gene. They put it off until some undefined point in the future, or they resolve to wait until they feel that something's physically wrong with them. Tragically, the first thing a person "feels" may be sudden death.

The Professor Who Almost Flunked the Test

Don, a 57-year-old university professor, had no outward symptoms of heart disease. But there were some significant "S.O.S." signals that showed up first on the treadmill stress test.

When he made his first visit to the Aerobics Center in 1981, he didn't seem to know it, but he was in lousy shape. His treadmill time was just ten minutes, a performance which put him in the "poor" fitness category for his age group. That wasn't surprising to us, because he was a bit overweight. But still, when we started the test, he had no outward symptoms of heart disease, and his resting ECG was normal. Also, his family history and blood pressure presented no cause for concern. A routine physical would have found no sign of trouble.

As he came to the end of the stress test, though, something happened to his ECG. An abnormal S-T segment appeared on a number of different leads. But still, I was cautious. Although there were several abnormalities, they were slight enough—just one millimeter off the usual course—to be considered an equivocal reading.

Unfortunately, my ability to evaluate Don's situation was limited because he had never taken a stress test before. He had always put it off. As a result, without any previous ECGs to compare this one to, we had no idea if the abnormality would remain stable, or if it was worsening. For all we knew, Don could have had heart readings like this for twenty years.

Since he didn't appear to be facing a life-threatening situation, we took no immediate action, other than to encourage him to change his lifestyle somewhat and lose weight. To his credit, Don took the advice. When he returned to the Clinic a few months later, he had lost twenty-seven pounds. Moreover, his treadmill time went from ten minutes up to fifteen minutes. So we moved his overall fitness classification up to "fair"—which was better, but still not all that terrific.

Most important, however, this time we noticed a more ominous sign of heart disease: Don's blood pressure dropped during the test. Also, his stress electrocardiogram showed an even greater abnormality in that all-important S-T segment. The line was off course by two millimeters.

The risk factors began to pile up against him. In fact, with this serious new change on his ECG, his risk profile became unacceptable. He now appeared to be a prime candidate for an imminent heart attack, so we immediately ordered a coronary arteriogram.

The test results were terrible. They showed astonishing amounts of fatty deposits clogging the vessels. One vessel was practically closed from arteriosclerosis. There was 90 to 95 percent obstruction in another vessel; it was almost totally choking it off. Still another major vessel was 90 percent blocked, and several others were more than 70 percent closed off.

Don checked into the hospital immediately. Within days, his surgeon performed a quintuple bypass. The surgeon confirmed that several blood vessels leading to key areas of the heart were virtually blocked and useless. Each one had the potential of wiping out a big segment of the heart, and perhaps killing him instantly.

By putting off his first stress test for so long, Don may have placed himself in serious jeopardy. During his last year before surgery, he was at needless risk of a heart attack. Had we been following his condition through regular stress tests, we might have been able to identify the problem earlier and take corrective action, which might have enabled him to avoid bypass surgery.

Because of remarkable results like these, I believe a regular maximal stress test, supervised by a knowledgeable physician, is advisable for everybody over forty. Now, I know that this statement may be a subject of controversy, due to costs, lack of available testing facilities, and all the other criticisms we've already considered. But as far as I'm concerned, if any suggestion or criticism is in order, it's that the stress tests must be improved and become more readily available for the masses.

It's true that some doctors have suggested stress tests should be limited only to those who show symptoms of heart disease or have major coronary risk factors. That may sound like a safe policy at first, but I really can't agree. Such an approach ignores the vast numbers of patients who showed no other symptoms and had minimal coronary risks, but for whom the test proved to be a lifesaver. As we just saw in Don's case, there was no chest pain and no other outward symptoms of disease. The stress test was the only obvious clue that something serious was wrong. Without such a test, it's quite possible that the man would have suffered a severe heart attack or even sudden death.

And remember: Don came to us when he was only slightly older than Jim Fixx. Like Fixx, he had progressive arteriosclerotic heart disease—even worse than what Fixx faced. Also like Fixx, he had virtually no symptoms. Yet *unlike* Fixx, Don began a program of regular evaluations. Consequently, Don was able to do something before he got that first and often fatal clue, a heart attack.

We've had thousands of patients with no symptoms whatsoever who have been screened at the Cooper Clinic—and who were found to have an abnormal stress test. So I would definitely have a hard time justifying the use of the stress test only for those who have symptoms, or who are known to have heart disease. We simply can't afford to fool around with coronary disease. Many people have been able to avoid painful coronary problems and are alive today because they went through this screening procedure.

But even as I sing the praises of the treadmill stress test, I want to be completely realistic. There's always room for improvement in the test, such as by minimizing false readings as much as possible. Recent developments in computer technology, for instance, seem especially promising.

In a recent study conducted at the Veterans Administration Medical Center and the University of California in San Francisco and also at the Walter Reed Army Medical Center, Dr. Milton Hollenberg and several colleagues used computers to analyze ECG results from treadmill stress tests.

Of the 377 young military officers tested, all of whom were without symptoms, there were less than 1 percent false-positive readings. Also, later coronary arteriography revealed that the one person whom the computerized approach predicted would have coronary artery disease, actually *did* have it. So it would seem that the future of the stress test is extremely bright.

But now, let's return to the present. In the next chapter, I'll introduce you to a stress test protocol that I believe, given our present state of knowledge and practice, can bring false readings to the lowest possible level for mass testing. Called the "Cooper Clinic Protocol," this procedure can be followed by any qualified person who conducts your stress test.

CHAPTER EIGHT

THE COOPER CLINIC PROTOCOL FOR A SAFE AND SENSITIVE STRESS TEST

Throughout this book, I've referred to the importance of stress testing for those who want to "run without fear." This test should also be a component part of any good preventive medical examination.

I believe that the Cooper Clinic Protocol (or in shortened form, Cooper Protocol) which we use for treadmill stress testing (TMST) makes that procedure as accurate as any noninvasive technique being used in cardiology today. Even though it's not foolproof, the test's accuracy, when done properly, makes it a very valuable diagnostic tool.

It combines state-of-the-art standards for evaluating cardiovascular fitness with the latest techniques for predicting the presence of heart disease. Because the procedures we are using are essentially a distillation of both the safest and most effective techniques in other stress test methods, they are under consideration for use by the U.S. Army and other testing centers.

We have tried to simplify certain techniques so that the stress test can become available to the widest segment of the public. As the

153

cornerstone of our own preventive medicine program, the Cooper Protocol also provides a step-by-step method of interpreting test results that may help to avoid unnecessary tests or surgery.

And you don't have to travel to the Aerobics Center in Dallas to take advantage of these benefits. Any qualified physician can use our basic test procedures to form the basis of a thorough exam. The testing equipment needed is readily available throughout the country.

So, for the next few pages, let's take a close look at the procedures that make up the Cooper Protocol. Medical professionals may want to refer to the detailed explanations of the Cooper Protocol in the Appendix. A chart summarizing information about the protocol also appears at the end of this chapter.

Here are the guidelines your physician or cardiac center should follow to conform to the Cooper Protocol when you go for your stress testing. I will attempt to present this from the patient's point of view so that the average lay reader will be in a better position to ask questions and understand his own test results.

Guideline #1:   Get a Thorough Pretest Screening

Before you even get on a treadmill, you must be evaluated to determine whether it is safe for you to have a maximal performance stress test. As I mentioned earlier, we try to be as careful as possible to avoid any risky procedures. These preliminary tests will tell your doctor whether you have any major medical problems and whether you are likely to have a false-positive stress electrocardiogram. By comparing this preliminary information to the stress test results, your doctor can better evaluate whether an abnormal test result might be a false positive or is truly abnormal.

Your initial screening should:

- include a brief history and physical examination, during which your physician listens to your heart and lungs;
- check for the use of drugs that are known to affect the electrocardiogram (e.g., various heart and hypertensive medications);

- check for a history of congenital or acquired heart disorders; and
- include a thorough evaluation of the resting ECG.

As to the last point, a proper screening procedure should include several resting ECGs. I recommend four twelve-lead ECGs.

To begin with, it's important to get two resting electrocardiograms with the electrodes in slightly different positions. The first is taken in the supine position—that is, while you are lying flat on your back. The electrodes are placed close to the ankles, wrists, and on the chest, in the positions used in taking a standard ECG.

The second ECG is also taken in the supine position, but with the electrodes placed in the location they will be in during the treadmill test. From the ankles, they are moved to the lower chest; from the wrists, they are moved to the collarbones.

A third resting ECG is taken while you're standing up. This is where an unsteady line—or "T-wave" inversion response—is often noted. Any irregularity at this stage is called a "postural response" and usually has nothing to do with coronary disease. But it's still an important reading because it gives your doctor valuable information to use when interpreting your final test results. For example, if an irregularity does appear at this stage, a positive stress ECG is more likely. And if this happens, it is very likely that it is a *false* positive.

Highly conditioned athletes, particularly distance runners, very commonly show this postural or T-wave response. In some of the medical literature, this is referred to as "the world-class athlete syndrome"; it's a common cause of a false-positive stress test. And remember: A false-positive test means that the ECG is abnormal but, in reality, no coronary artery disease exists.

The fourth ECG should be taken after hyperventilation, which involves breathing deeply and rapidly for a period of at least twenty seconds. Abnormal ECGs that occur during hyperventilation are a cause of false positives, which again, are commonly found in highly conditioned endurance athletes. False positives are also most often found in women, who historically have a higher incidence than do men.

This fourth resting ECG is very important in helping your doctor determine whether a positive reading during the exercise phase of your test is a false or true positive.

Guideline #2: Monitor a Minimum of Nine ECG Leads, with Seven Chest Electrodes

For an accurate test, you must have at least seven electrodes attached to your chest. This enables the person conducting the test to monitor nine ECG leads.

At the Cooper Clinic, we monitor fifteen leads, using fourteen electrodes. (See Figure 1.) Some researchers believe this many is unnecessary, but our experience indicates otherwise. We've discovered that your chances of getting truer readings on the ECG improve if more electrodes are used. In most hospitals and testing laboratories, ten electrodes are used. This approach, which permits the monitoring of a standard twelve-lead ECG, is adequate.

In any event, check to see whether *at least* seven electrodes are being used to monitor your heart during the test. Do not accept a three- or five-electrode method, because they are not adequate and may lull you into a false sense of security if your test turns out to be normal. (See Figure 2.)

Guideline #3: Use the Proper Treadmill Procedure

I say "treadmill" because I believe the treadmill test is superior to either bicycle testing or the Masters two-step test. But even with the treadmill, there are different protocols that can be used.

For example, the test most commonly used is the Bruce Protocol. In this test, both the speed and the incline of the treadmill are increased every three minutes. (See Figure 3.)

On the other hand, the test I prefer is a modified version of the Balke Protocol. With the Balke method, the speed is held constant at 3.3 m.p.h. (90 meters per minute) until the twenty-fifth minute, at which time it is increased 0.2 m.p.h. each minute. The treadmill is flat the first minute, and then increases by 2 percent. Each minute thereafter, it is increased one percent per minute until the twenty-fifth minute. After that, only the speed increases; the incline remains at 25 percent. (See Figure 4.)

Although it takes longer to perform the Balke than the Bruce test, the Balke provides more of a warm-up and usually does not require running. I believe these differences make the Balke test safer.

Figure 1.

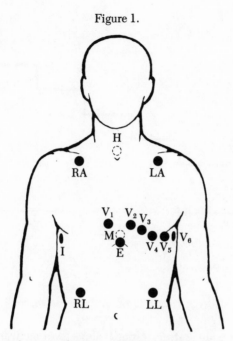

Fifteen Lead System of Electrode Placement

Figure 2.

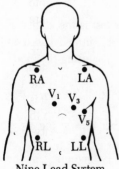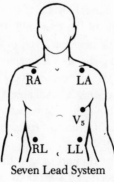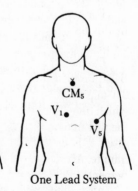

Nine Lead System Seven Lead System One Lead System

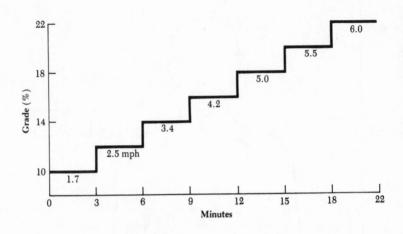

Figure 3. Bruce Protocol

To convert Bruce treadmill times to the Balke, multiply the time in minutes by 1.75.

Regular treadmill stress testing is also a great motivation tool. We have age- and sex-adjusted test records at the Cooper Clinic, which represent the best performances in more than 60,000 tests. Moreover, even though a patient may not be able to establish a clinic record, just the act of documenting personal improvement can be highly motivational. We've found that this helps the patients to maintain their goals and often improve their fitness level.

Another valuable role of the treadmill stress test is the ability of an individual to determine personal levels of aerobic fitness, based on sex and age. All of these goals are easily achieved by using the modified Balke method with the Cooper Protocol.

Whatever form of testing is available to you, there are a few elements of proper treadmill procedure that you should keep in mind.

First of all, don't hold onto the treadmill bar during the stress test.

Hold onto the bar for support only at the very beginning, as the treadmill increases in speed and your body adjusts to the movement and balance required. You should hold onto the bar only for a minute, or a minute and a half at the maximum. Afterwards, as you move into

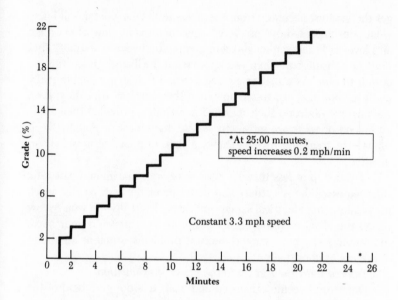

Figure 4. Balke Protocol

a steady pace during this early, submaximal phase of your workout, you should let your arms swing freely.

Many times, I've seen the exercising heart rate drop when a patient grabs hold of the bar during the treadmill stress test. The problem with this is that the energy requirement decreases when you hold onto the bar. At times, of course, it's necessary to grab hold because the patient becomes unstable. But in such cases, the level of aerobic fitness can't be determined accurately. Regardless of whether you hold onto the bar or not, testing for coronary disease is possible, however, provided the age-adjusted, fitness-adjusted maximal heart rate is reached.

Second, keep exercising to your maximum heart rate.

This is just a continuation of the discussion we started above. As we've seen, you may keep yourself from reaching your maximum heart rate simply by holding onto the treadmill bar. But you may also fail to achieve that level if you allow yourself to give up too soon.

Hitting that maximum heart rate is important to enable you to get the greatest accuracy from the stress test. Your doctor will know what your expected or "predicted" maximum is in view of your age and level of fitness, although there is some individual variability that must be considered. When you approach it, he'll start giving you the option to quit. As a matter of fact, we find that many people really *want* to continue, just to see how long they can last. I let them keep walking even beyond their maximal heart rates, provided their ECG and blood pressure are satisfactory. Also, they must be able to "keep up" on the treadmill without showing signs of a lack of muscle coordination.

If you stop at less than 85 percent of your maximum heart rate, that decreases the sensitivity and accuracy of the test. At that level, it's possible that electrical signals indicating heart disease won't show up on the ECG monitor. So it's desirable to exercise to your maximum unless you have some significant problems—such as an abnormal ECG or chest pain.

Proceed with the test up to the point of exhaustion.

Once you become exhausted and want to stop, grab hold of the bar, and the cool-down procedure will begin.

By exhaustion, I mean that point when you start to get markedly fatigued. Probably, you'll start having some difficulty in keeping up with the pace of the treadmill; or you'll become so winded that you can't talk while you're exercising. You may even have some symptoms, such as chest tightness. This point is what we refer to as "symptom-limited maximum performance."

I recall when I first stress-tested my wife several years ago. I told her that I wanted her to exercise to the point of exhaustion.

"How will I know when I've become exhausted?" she asked.

"You'll know," was my response.

During the final few minutes of her maximal performance test, she had to combine walking and jogging just to keep up with the treadmill, and she became so winded that she could barely respond to questions.

After she finished the test and was about to dismount from the treadmill, I asked, "Did you know when you were exhausted?"

"There wasn't a question in my mind!" she said, as she staggered off the machine.

Allow yourself three to five minutes of low-intensity walking immediately following maximal performance.

This is the cool-down phase of the treadmill test. It's just as important as the cool-down after regular aerobic exercise. Above all, you should not stop suddenly. Rather, once you reach exhaustion, the incline should immediately be taken out of the treadmill. Ideally, it should be returned to a flat plane within fifteen to twenty seconds. At the same time, the treadmill speed drops from 3.3 to 2.2 miles per hour, and then to 1.5 to 2.2 miles per hour. At that speed, you should continue walking for the next three to five minutes. Following a normal test, three minutes is adequate, but five minutes is required after an abnormal test.

Finally, lie down.

You deserve it! In this recovery phase, you should "float over" to the exam table and lie flat on your back for a minimum of ten minutes of recovery. During this time, your blood pressure and ECG should be monitored at two to three minute intervals until they have returned to normal.

I have followed this protocol for stress testing in more than 70,000 maximal performance stress tests during the past twenty years. As I've said before, I've never had a death associated with stress testing. Furthermore, our sensitivity in identifying coronary artery disease with stress testing exceeds 80 percent. So stress testing *can* be safe and effective—if it's done properly!

Guideline #4: Ask Your Doctor for a Blood Evaluation

If your stress test is abnormal, blood studies may provide further information as to the severity of the problem. For example, they may show a high fat content in your blood, or an unhealthy total cholesterol/HDL cholesterol ratio (i.e., more than 5.0 for men or more than 4.5 for women).

In the not-too-distant future, we may even be able to ask our doctors routinely for the levels of smaller components of our HDLs, namely HDL-2 and HDL-3 readings. Also, the levels of another substance, "apolipoprotein B," may be the best indicator of arteriosclerosis, particularly among relatives of patients with proven heart disease. (For further information on these points, see P. O. Kwiterovich, Johns

Hopkins Medical School, American Public Health Association Meeting, Anaheim, California, 1984; G. L. Vega and S. M. Grundy, "Comparison of Apolipoprotein B to Cholesterol in Low Density Lipoproteins of Patients with Coronary Heart Disease," *Journal of Lipid Research,* Vol. 25, 1984.) But for now, these tests are very experimental and expensive, and they are limited primarily to use in research laboratories.

These are the guidelines your doctor should use in conducting a stress test according to the Cooper Protocol. Now, what are some of the specific things we can learn from such a stress test?

As I mentioned in an earlier chapter, evaluating stress tests may be a judgment call; in other words, there is some room for doubt and interpretation. But still, it's not just a hit-or-miss affair. The type of treatment recommended is always based on the best evidence we have available, as documented in the medical literature. Also, to ensure we don't begin to rely on isolated or unsupported findings, we tend to be conservative in the treatment we recommend.

For example, under no circumstances would we rush people in for a coronary arteriogram or some other such test at the first sign of an abnormal ECG. That may be the policy of some physicians, but most, like us, would be much more conservative. Even a long-term history of an abnormal stress ECG or a personal history of heart disease does not necessarily place a patient at risk of an imminent heart attack.

Instead, we've learned after years of experience that there may be an extremely wide variety of heart conditions in different people. As a result, we now try to *classify* various coronary problems and treatments in order to give a person the safest and most personal care. In the interest of avoiding unnecessary treatment and surgery, the Cooper Protocol has been designed to fine-tune the evaluation process. We recommend treatment only when a person is clearly in danger of having a major heart problem. It's quite possible, after all, that an abnormal heart condition could stay stable for many years, and present no danger.

In one 59-year-old man named Richard, for instance, we tracked an abnormal heart condition for eight years following an acute heart attack in 1974. When he first came to the Cooper Clinic in January 1975, Richard lasted only thirteen minutes on the treadmill, and that placed him in the "poor" fitness category. Overall, his risk profile showed that he was at a "high" level of risk.

For one thing, the electrocardiogram taken during his first stress test was abnormal. Also, there was a family history of coronary heart disease because his brother died at an early age from a heart attack. He had been a smoker; he worked in a moderately tense environment; he was overweight; and finally, he had elevated levels of blood fats.

Still, there was no indication of any immediate danger, and his condition seemed to have stabilized. In particular, despite his heart attack, he was completely without symptoms, both at rest and while exercising.

Richard returned to our Clinic every year, and though his stress ECGs continued to be abnormal, his treadmill time steadily improved. By January 1983, he was up to nineteen minutes, an effort that placed him in the "excellent" fitness category for his age. He was having no discomfort or outward symptoms, and his resting ECG was still equivocal.

But during this 1983 exam, some new and extremely important danger signals emerged: Richard's stress ECG was grossly abnormal.

Our approach in cases like this is clear. Because of the obvious alteration or "serial change" in his electrocardiogram, we recommended that he undergo a coronary arteriogram. As it happened, the test was conducted just in time. Although Richard was still without symptoms, the coronary arteriogram revealed almost total blockage in several major vessels. He could have had a heart attack at any time.

Within days, Richard had a multiple-vessel coronary bypass operation, and today, he's doing well. But as you can see, we didn't rush into surgery. Even though there were a number of danger signals that appeared on his stress tests and elsewhere in his medical exam, we waited for a clear sign that his condition had deteriorated. In fact, Richard did very well for eight years. It was only when the danger to his life and health became obvious by a serial change in his electrocardiogram that we recommended additional testing.

So that cases like this can be handled intelligently and sensitively, the physician interpreting the stress electrocardiogram must make valid decisions at the time of the stress test. Now, let's explore what information various stress test results may convey to your physician and how to handle these different types of problems.

Normal

Even if your stress test is normal, you shouldn't get complacent. If you're over forty years old, you should schedule another stress test at *least* every three years. Better still, I would strongly advise you to get one every year. A single, normal stress test in no way means life-long immunity to heart disease, and it is an excellent way to quantify your current level of fitness. The Appendix contains age-adjusted fitness categories for men and women as determined by treadmill time.

Normal, but Signs of "Exertional Angina"

In this case, you have a normal stress electrocardiogram, but you notice some chest pain when you are approaching your maximum capacity. By definition, chest pain that occurs with exercise always categorizes a stress test as being abnormal, regardless of the results of the ECG. Also, a drop in heart rate or systolic blood pressure in the presence of an increasing work load is considered to be abnormal. It's best to reevaluate these patients with another test in three to six months.

Normal, but "Poor Responder"

By a "poor responder," I'm referring to those people who feel they *must* quit shortly after the test begins, even though the heart rate has still not been appreciably elevated. The ECG is completely normal, but the test would have to be classified as inconclusive, if not abnormal.

Because there could be some serious coronary artery disease that the stress test isn't picking up at submaximal levels of exercise, we recommend that these people enroll in a medically supervised progressive exercise program. Also, they should be reevaluated within three months after their level of fitness has improved.

Athletic Normal

People whom we classify in this category have an abnormal resting ECG (usually T-wave inversion in leads II, III, AVF, V_{3-6}—see Figure 5), but all the abnormalities disappear during exercise. Follow-

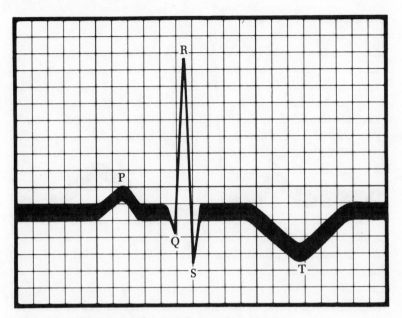

Figure 5. ECG Tracing Showing T-wave Inversion

up studies have shown that these people usually are not really at any increased risk of heart attack.

Equivocal

When we start seeing equivocal readings on the ECG, that means that some abnormalities are beginning to show up on the test. (See Figure 6.) Ordinarily, though, they are not severe enough to cause too much concern. Some congenital heart disorders can cause this, as can early arteriosclerosis. Typically, we ask people with this kind of reading to get additional studies, sometimes including an echocardiogram.

In follow-up studies of patients with equivocal stress tests, I've noticed that the ECG can do one of three things: remain the same; revert to a normal response; or progress to the point where it is clearly abnormal. Many times, what happens with the electrocardio-

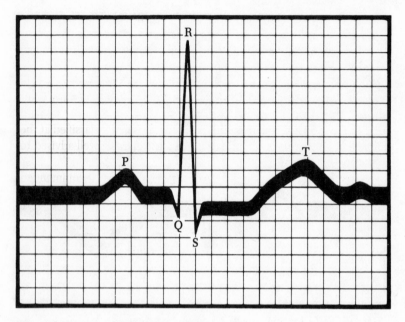

Figure 6. Equivocal S-T Segment Response

gram depends on what the patient does in his or her rehabilitation program.

Abnormal

With all the different types of "normal" readings that I've just mentioned, you have probably already guessed that there are a number of abnormal readings as well. Surprisingly, many doctors and researchers simply lump all positive stress tests into one general category—abnormal. But as I'll show you, we can be more precise than that. In fact, to get more reliable test results, a physician *must* dig deeper into the facts of each individual case than just to attach the broad label "abnormal."

In our classification system, there are several different degrees or "levels" we have established for the positive or abnormal stress test.

Not all of them are life-threatening, but each does require a different kind of follow-up.

For the first two levels, a doctor may just tell you to return in three to six months for more monitoring. In this way, he can observe your progress and can respond immediately if the abnormality in your stress test begins to get worse. At these early levels, we don't ordinarily suggest additional studies.

But, as you'll see on the next few pages, if you are classified at the more extreme levels of abnormality, then you may be well-advised to get some additional studies.

Any of the following five basic studies may be recommended after an abnormal stress test:

• *Blood studies.* The doctor may order additional special reports from the laboratory on certain key components in your blood, such as your lipid levels or cardiac enzymes. It's always advisable to have screening blood studies done in conjunction with your stress test. But after the test, your physician may want to double-check some readings or order additional studies.

• *Echocardiogram.* This involves using high-frequency sound waves to provide a picture of the heart. It's especially helpful in detecting congenital defects, such as the enlarged and abnormal heart that Jim Fixx had.

• *Holter monitoring.* This sophisticated procedure requires making a recording on magnetic tape of the heart's electrical signals, as they are emitted during an electrocardiogram over a twenty-four-hour period. Then, the signals are replayed and scanned in an effort to pick up important but fleeting changes that might slip through undetected in an ordinary electrocardiogram.

• *MUGA scan.* This is an acronym standing for multiple-gated acquisition. It's a specialized test that involves checking the condition of the heart through techniques still being developed in the new science of nuclear medicine.

A thallium scan is another radioisotopic technique being used to diagnose obstructive coronary-artery disease. Its reliability and accuracy are debated, however, and some investigators feel it has little to add to treadmill testing. As we discussed earlier, I had one case where the thallium scan was normal. But because the person had an abnormal stress test, I requested a coronary arteriogram. That test revealed multiple-vessel disease, and a life-saving bypass procedure was performed.

• *Coronary arteriogram.* As you already know, this procedure, perhaps the most conclusive test in detecting clogged coronary arteries, requires the insertion of a catheter through the femoral artery in the groin. The catheter is then pushed up into the coronary arteries, and an X-ray is taken as a radio-opaque dye is injected into the arteries. This test shows the exact degree of blockage.

These, then, are some of the further tests that may be ordered if you have an abnormal stress test. Now, with this background in mind, let's see how various stress-test abnormalities are classified to determine which, if any, of these additional tests are appropriate. As you read through these classifications, you might also want to refer to these charts in the Appendix: the absolute contraindications to stress testing, and the ways to handle treadmill abnormalities.

Abnormal Level One

The stress test is abnormal only during the final few minutes of a true maximum performance. The patient has a normal resting and recovery phase.

It's possible that some coronary disease exists here, but if it does, it's probably not too serious. The outlook is about the same as for a normal stress-test response. No specific treatment or additional studies are required. The only recommendation we would make is that you have another stress test within six months, rather than wait a full year.

Abnormal Level Two

The stress test is abnormal at submaximal levels, but normal at maximal. Also, it's normal or equivocal at resting and recovery.

Most likely, this result is not an indication of coronary disease. It could be related to the presence of drugs, such as those used for treating hypertension. An electrolyte deficiency such as low potassium can also cause such a change, as can vasoregulatory phenomena. Or it might arise from some congenital heart disorder. To be on the safe side, we usually recommend that additional blood studies be made to give us a more complete picture of your overall coronary risk. If the results of these tests are normal, the only other recommendation would be another stress test within six months.

Abnormal Level Three

The stress test is normal during the exercise portion of the test. Abnormality develops only during recovery.

In this case, it's very likely that there is some coronary disease, though it may not be serious. Depending on the magnitude of the abnormality that emerges on the ECG, additional studies may be required. In most cases, though, we would just recommend that you return for another evaluation in six to twelve months.

Abnormal Level Four

Stress test is normal at rest and at submaximal exercise levels. But it becomes abnormal during maximal exertion and persists through recovery.

This kind of abnormal reading could result from a wide range of disorders. If you are using drugs for hypertension or heart disease, for example, or if you have a congenital heart problem, an ECG could show a false positive. But it could also result from genuine coronary obstructive disease.

We would recommend additional blood studies, and in some cases, an echocardiogram. You should also come back to be reevaluated with another stress test within six months.

Abnormal Level Five

The ECG is normal at rest, but during exercise it becomes abnormal. The abnormality then persists through maximum exertion, and into recovery.

Most times, the only reason for this pattern of abnormality is serious arteriosclerosis, or the classic hardening of the arteries that afflicted Jim Fixx. Because this can be a dangerous condition, we would recommend a series of additional studies. These might include extra blood studies and perhaps an echocardiogram. Depending upon the results of these tests, the Holter monitoring or MUGA scan mentioned above might also be performed.

The scheduling of another stress test will depend upon the results of these studies. Generally, a follow-up stress test should be taken within three to six months, unless the additional tests are clearly abnormal. In such a case, coronary arteriography would be recommended.

Abnormal Level Six

This final, most serious indication of abnormality on a stress test shows an unusual resting ECG pattern which persists into submaximal exercise. A major abnormality then develops before the maximum heart rate is reached, and the patient must be stopped during exercise. The abnormality continues through recovery. Angina may or may not be present in such cases.

This degree of abnormality during a stress test typically indicates severe coronary obstructive disease. Blood studies and echocardiograms are often ordered, but in most cases they are accompanied by a coronary arteriogram. If the test results show that immediate treatment isn't necessary, then a reevaluation on a treadmill within three months should be scheduled.

Even with this variety of abnormal categories, it's not always clear into just what level a given person's test may fall. As more research continues to be reported, we constantly modify our interpretations.

As I mentioned in the last chapter, when the stress ECG changes from one test to the next, that is often a good indication of heart disease. In the past, when our knowledge was more limited, many doctors would have ignored these changes if the patient had no chest pain or other cardiac symptoms.

But now we know that even in highly conditioned marathoners, a major, serial change in the stress ECG can point to some serious underlying problem. We sometimes recommend a coronary arteriogram for such patients.

In my experience, *any* change in the status of the ECG is often a key confirmation of a patient's deteriorating condition. But unless a person has regular stress tests, his doctor might miss that crucial turning point when the patient's condition becomes more dangerous and he begins to face a much higher risk of a heart attack.

No matter who you are or what your other risk factors seem to be saying, you can never rely on your lack of symptoms. Even an active, athletic person may suddenly be at great risk of a coronary event and never even realize it. Without an electrocardiogram taken under exercise conditions, he may never know the true state of his health until the first symptom develops. And that first outward symptom may be sudden death.

On the other hand, regular monitoring of these changes has helped us save many lives. For instance, Jim, an athletic 47-year-old orthodontist, started having an annual stress test in July 1972. At that time, he was in excellent condition: He could walk twenty-two minutes on the treadmill, and he had a normal resting and stress ECG. On his annual visits in subsequent years, he retained his good time on the treadmill and kept his level of fitness in the "excellent" category.

But then, in August 1982, a change developed in his stress test. His maximum heart rate dropped to 148 beats per minute. While a decrease in heart rate is normal with age, this sudden drop went far beyond what was usual.

Jim's blood pressure also was elevated, and the fats in his blood were unusually high. So we placed him on medications to lower his lipid abnormality and to bring his hypertension back into line. Also, we asked him to return for a six-month follow-up, rather than the usual annual test.

When he returned, his treadmill stress test was much worse and now grossly abnormal: He lasted only thirteen minutes on the treadmill, with some chest discomfort at the eleven-minute mark. And on his ECG, for the first time, there was a classic abnormality that we noted at rest, during exercise, and during recovery.

As far as other risk factors were concerned, there was known coronary disease in his family. His sister had died of a heart attack at age forty-five, and his father had a first heart attack at age fifty-five. Also, Jim was a smoker, lived under a high level of tension, had borderline hypertension, and showed extremely high levels of blood fats in his blood studies.

His overall coronary risk until this last test, though, had been considered moderate. But with the new information from the stress test he went into the high-risk range and had to be classified at the sixth, or highest, level of abnormality.

Given all the danger signs we had picked up, we ordered a coronary arteriogram. The news wasn't good. One blood vessel was 90 percent obstructed, and two others were about 70 percent clogged. He had a triple-vessel bypass operation, from which he recovered rapidly. I'm happy to say that as this book goes to print, Jim has returned to regular workouts under our supervision at the Aerobics Center. Also, he is without symptoms, and his stress test is normal.

Perhaps the most important lesson to learn from this illustration is that this dentist had never shown any symptoms of heart disease until his *last* stress test.

As you can see, coronary disease can progress quickly, once it begins. In this particular case, Jim's condition deteriorated markedly in just six months' time. But because we monitored him so closely with frequent check-ups and stress tests, we were able to respond appropriately before any major damage had occurred.

Finally, there is sometimes an ultimate success story we can tell about our stress tests. On occasion, the results of a properly administered stress test actually seem able to help us *reverse* the course of coronary artery disease. In particular, a reversal can happen if a person's condition has been abnormal for a period that's as short as four to six months.

Take the situation of a vice president of a large local company who came to us in November 1983 for a stress test. Although he was considerably overweight at 197 pounds, he had been exercising regularly and managed to go for twenty minutes on the treadmill—a performance which ranked him in the "excellent" category of fitness for a man fifty-three years old. But there were some problems.

When he reached his maximum heart rate, his ECG was grossly abnormal, even though at all other times the ECG was relatively normal. Also, his cholesterol and triglycerides were elevated, and his overall coronary risk was high by our predictive standards.

So we classified him at Abnormal Level One. At that level, it was likely that there was some obstructive disease, but it was probably minimal. As a result, it wasn't necessary for us to take any extreme measures of treatment. Instead, we put him into a rehabilitation program, which involved cutting his calories and changing his eating habits.

He responded wonderfully to the program. When he came back to the Clinic in March 1984, just four months after his previous stress test, he had lost twenty-four pounds. Then came the real test: He got onto the treadmill—rather confidently, I thought. As he passed the twenty-minute mark, we watched the monitors carefully for signs of his previous trouble. But there was none. He ran past twenty-one, then twenty-two minutes without a hitch. We were astonished when he finally pooped out at twenty-four minutes, a full four minutes longer than the mark he had reached just four months earlier!

In addition to his weight loss, this man's cholesterol and triglycerides were way down. On the treadmill stress test, his ECG was now normal all the way through. And he continued to improve in succeeding months. By November 1984 he had established his all-time record on the treadmill—twenty-seven minutes.

The explanation for this dramatic turn-around? Fortunately, we had been able to catch his disease at a point where we could reverse the abnormality. And he greatly improved his long-term chances of survival.

Such cases show why it's so important to do regular stress testing, even on seemingly normal people who show no symptoms. By following the guidelines that I've outlined in this chapter, you may be able to catch heart disease before those first symptoms strike. And if you catch the disease early enough, you may even be able to reverse a life-threatening condition.

Refining our Cooper Protocol won't stop here, of course. As time goes on, more and more research will show us other ways to adapt the treadmill procedure and to evaluate the test results. For example, recent research shows an important correlation between S-T segment depression and heart rate. Some researchers suggest that comparing these two factors may be one of the most accurate ways yet to detect disease. We'll continue to watch these and other developments, and fine-tune our procedures accordingly.

So, as future studies bring other facts to light, we'll develop even more effective tools for evaluating our tests and reducing the risk of coronary disease. And as you'll see in the next chapter, these new testing procedures may even move us closer to a goal that has tantalized medical experts for ages—they may help us prolong your life.

COOPER CLINIC PROTOCOL
Diagnosis, Management and Recommendations for Re-evaluation

TREADMILL STRESS TEST — 7 or more electrodes — Maximum Performance — Bruce or Balke Protocol	Normal Stress ECG (N)
	Normal Stress ECG but exertional chest pain
	Normal Stress ECG but poor responder (exhausted at low heart rate)
	Athletic Normal (ECG abnormal at rest, normal with exercise)
	Equivocal Stress ECG

Abnormal Stress ECG (Abn)

	Rest	Submax	Max	Recover.
I	N	N	Abn#	N
II	N	Abn	N	N
III	N	N	N	Abn
IV	N	N	Abn	Abn
V	N	Abn	Abn	Abn
VI	Abn	Abn##	—	Abn

#Only during the final 2:00 of a
max performance test. If coronary
disease, it is not significant

##Stopped at low heart rates due to
abnormal ECG. Very likely it is
severe coronary disease

Diagnosis:
NV—Normal Variant
R_X—(Digitalis, Diuretics, B-blockers, Quinidine, Sedatives, etc.)
BP—Hypertensive response with exercise
El—Electrolyte deficiency (hypokalemia)
T—T-wave lability (postural or hyperventilation response)
Val—Valvular Disease (aortic stenosis or mitral valve prolapse)
CD—Conduction defects (CLBBB, CRBBB)
My—Myocardial Disease (LVH, IHSS, ASH, HCM, Cor. artery
     bridging, Old MI, Cor. spasm.
CAD—Obstructive Coronary Disease

Diagnosis or Cause	Management*	Treadmill Stress Test Re-evaluation Frequency
Normal	None Required	>40 years, at least every 3 years
Probable CAD	B, CM, SCR, Ec Possibly CA	3 months
Possible CAD	B, SCR	3-6 months
NV	Reassurance; B, X, As	<40 years, every 3 years >40 years, every year
All diagnoses listed	B, X, As, DE	6-12 months
NV, BP, El, Val, ?CAD	Reassurance, B, As, X	12 months
NV, R_X, El, Val, My	B, As, X, Ec, DE	12 months
BP, El, T, ? CAD	B, As, X, DE	6 months
R_X, BP, El, Val, My, CAD	B, As, X, Ec, ? HM, MTS	6 months (in SCR)
El, My, Probable CAD	B, As, X, Ec, HM MTS, or CA	3-6 months (in SCR)
Probable CAD	B, As, X, MTS, CA	3 months

Management decisions depend not only on laboratory and ECG results, but also on clinical judgement, family history, body weight, fitness level, smoking history, etc. One or more of the suggested studies may be performed depending upon the results of a study and/or the magnitude of the abnormality.

Management:
B—Blood studies incl. lipids
As—Chest auscultation
X—Chext x-ray
Ec—Echocardiogram
HM—24 hr. Holter Monitoring
MTS — MUGA or thallium scan
CA—Coronary Arteriogram
CM—Cardiac R_X
SCR—Supervised cardiac rehab
DE—Diet and exercise program, no supervision

CHAPTER NINE

CAN YOU REALLY PROLONG YOUR LIFE?

One of the memories that I have of a very old friend of mine is the way she read the newspaper. She'd turn to her favorite section and then chuckle. Then, she'd read some more and chuckle even louder.

You might think the part of the paper that was giving her so much pleasure was the comics, but that wasn't it. She was reading the obituary page.

She'd check the ages of each of the deceased and take great pride in the number of people she had outlived. She thought of herself as a very lucky woman because she had enjoyed such a long and healthy life. And she wasn't really being morbid. Rather, she was just feeling good about herself and the level of energy she still retained.

Most people may not get so much of a kick out of the obituary page. But it's easy to appreciate this elderly woman's sense of satisfaction about reaching a ripe old age, especially since she had managed to stay quite active and healthy. In fact, she had reached one of the ultimate goals that human beings hope for—a spry, productive, and very long life span.

People have always looked for ways to prolong their lives and preserve their youth. Since the dawn of time, human beings have searched for an elixir of eternal youth and health. In less sophisticated days, some believed in the possibility of the sorcerer's potion, rumored to have the power to turn back the clock of life. Such superstitions are reflected in the legends surrounding King Arthur's half-demon court magician, Merlin.

The quest became more concrete when a certain fifteenth-century adventurer sailed with Columbus on his second voyage to the Americas in 1493. This 33-year-old Spanish officer, Juan Ponce de Leon, soon rose to the governorship of "Porto Rico" in the West Indies. And along the way, he became enthralled with an Indian legend of an island called "Bimini." In this fabled land, a marvelous natural spring was supposed to flow with waters that could cure deadly disease and even bestow on the old their long-lost youth.

Ponce de Leon made such a convincing case to the Spanish authorities about the existence of this island that he secured a royal grant to discover and settle it. He failed to find Bimini, of course. But in the process of his explorations he did discover Florida, which in an ironic twist was to become a major haven for the aged and retired of a later time.

Despite such false starts, the search for eternal youth—or at least for an extended period of energetic life and health—has continued up to our own time. Within the last century, the wealthy in search of their lost youth have been known to frequent fancy, private clinics for unborn lamb or monkey gland treatments.

We're now discovering, however, that there's no need simply to chase such fantasies. Instead, the best approach is to work vigorously in our medical labs and testing facilities to conquer disease. Also, we can encourage lifestyles that lay the groundwork for greater longevity.

There are even some concrete signs that the first trickles of a "Spring of Youth" have already begun to reach us—though not in quite the way that the seekers of Bimini envisioned. During the decade of the 1970s, Americans enjoyed nearly a four-year increase in their average life expectancy—a surge that was almost four times the increase in life span for any previous decade. Furthermore, some health pundits predict that the average American woman will live to age ninety by the end of this century, and the average man to the mid-eighties. Most exciting of all, many experts feel that this trend toward a more advanced age can be accompanied by vim and vigor. ("Hope Grows for Vigorous Old Age," *The New York Times,* October 2, 1984.)

What exactly are the reasons that we can expect such progress in increasing our longevity?

The answer is actually rather simple: The two major causes of death in the United States are heart disease and cancer, in that order. If you can reduce your risk of suffering or dying from these two, then you greatly enhance your chances of a long life.

It's quite true that we have made great strides in blunting the threat posed by these two killers. Yet, they still remain the major reasons that most people in more advanced societies don't live longer. So what can you do in your own personal health program to enhance your chances of avoiding death and living to a ripe old age?

I believe there are four basic "Longevity Habits" which can reduce the chances the average person will suffer early death—and that means sudden *or* lingering death. If you make these practices part of your daily existence, you'll almost certainly add years to your life. These Longevity Habits include the following:

Habit #1: Have regular preventive medical exams, with adequate cardiovascular and cancer screening tests.

Habit #2: Eat a low-fat, low-sugar, low-salt, high-fiber diet, which will keep your weight within normal limits.

Habit #3: Follow a moderate but systematic aerobic exercise program.

Habit #4: Avoid tobacco in all forms, but particularly avoid cigarette smoking.

These four habits are designed to achieve several key objectives. Specifically:

- The preventive health exams help to identify heart disease and cancer at the earliest possible moment.
- A healthy diet, intelligent exercise program, and no-smoking commitment will reduce the threat of major killers such as arteriosclerosis, hypertension, obesity, unhealthy cholesterol levels in the blood, sedentary living, and cancer.
- Finally, even if you've suffered from a heart attack or other coronary problem, these Longevity Habits can help you return to good health through a cardiac rehabilitation program.

Now, I realize that there are many other risk factors and threats to life and limb that I haven't mentioned in these four Longevity Habits. Some of these additional concerns have been included in the earlier chapter in this book describing the Rules of Risk. There are also many others we haven't even considered in this book, such as the abuse of alcohol or the addiction to habit-forming drugs, which can cut anyone's life short in a variety of ways.

But if asked to select a few easy-to-remember rules of thumb that would lengthen the lives of the majority of people, I'd still settle on these four habits. They are the keys to increased longevity, though most of us, in one way or another, have unfortunately failed to make them a part of our lives.

And one other thing: It's absolutely essential that you follow *all* of these Longevity Habits if you hope to prolong your life. Just doing one, two, or three won't do the trick. Take Jim Fixx. He did a great job incorporating the last three habits into his daily routine for the last fifteen or so years of his life. But he omitted the first—the need for an annual health exam with a stress test. That omission probably led him down the road to sudden death.

With this general background about longevity in mind, I want to consider some specifics about the relationship between longevity and exercise. Here are a number of questions that I often hear on this issue, with my responses to each.

Question #1: Can Exercise Prolong My Life?

At the present time, we have many studies that strongly suggest life can *probably* be prolonged through a systematic, moderate aerobic exercise program. By "moderate," I mean the equivalent of my recommended four-times-a-week, twenty to thirty minute jogging sessions, covering a total of twelve to fifteen miles per week. Other aerobic exercises requiring comparable energy expenditure are equally as effective.

But right now, no one can state flatly that regular exercise definitely will increase the life span—and for a very good reason: To demonstrate that any particular factor prolongs life, we'd need studies covering the entire life spans of exercisers and nonexercisers. Such studies have been started, but the final results aren't in yet.

On the other hand, shorter-term studies have been done by such researchers as Dr. Ralph Paffenbarger and Dr. J. N. Morris. Both indicate that sedentary men are more susceptible to heart disease than are active men.

The Paffenbarger study, which centered on San Francisco long-shoremen, covered a period of some twenty years. During this re-search, Paffenbarger discovered that the men with jobs that required the most physical demands were least likely to die of heart problems. The same held true in the Morris study, which showed that the con-ductors on British double-deck buses, who did a lot of stair-climbing, lived longer than the drivers, who mainly sat during the workday.

Probably no single study correlating physical activity, coronary disease and longevity has been more debated than this 1953 study. Three years later, even Morris and his co-workers repudiated their original conclusions, stating that the conductors and drivers were really not similar people from the outset of the study. (See the 1956 article in Volume 2 of the British publication *Lancet*, pp. 566–570.) Specifically, it seems that the bus drivers were fatter than the conduc-tors, even at the time they were first hired; their girth and weight were greater.

From this 1956 article, one might believe that Morris didn't feel that exercise was a factor in preventing coronary disease. Yet he continued his research, and twenty-four years later, published an arti-cle entitled "Vigorous Exercise in Leisure Time: Protection Against Coronary Heart Disease" (*Lancet* 1980, 2:1207–1210). The title seems to speak for itself, and in the article, Professor Morris states: "Vigorous exercise is a natural defense of the body, with a protective effect on the aging heart against ischaemia and its consequences."

The Paffenbarger longshoreman study has also been debated. But Dr. Paffenbarger has continued his methodical research and, in July 1984, he reported on 16,936 Harvard alumni, whom he followed from 1962 to 1978. In this investigation, he found that those who engaged in regular exercise had one-half the death rate from heart disease as those who didn't exercise routinely. This was the first large, longitudi-nal study which showed that regular exercise *does* prolong life. (See the *Journal of the American Medical Association*, July 27, 1984, Vol. 252, No. 4.)

As yet, we don't have any completed studies that focus on people who change from inactivity to regular exercise in their middle years. But some research projects are now in progress. I expect they'll eventually provide strong evidence that exercise prevents or delays the onset of heart disease, and thereby reduces the risk of sudden death and enhances longevity.

Question #2:   Does Regular Exercise Shorten Life?

The exercise antagonist will say that running shortened Jim Fixx's life. The exercise enthusiast, on the other hand, will argue that it enabled him to live nine years longer than his father.

Realistically, no conclusions of this sort can be drawn from isolated examples. But there's another way of approaching this question. If exercise does shorten the life span, however, it seems logical that our average national life span should have decreased as the number of adults in the United States who exercise increased from 24 percent in 1961 to 59 percent in 1984. But the opposite occurred. Since 1961, the American life span has steadily increased by more than five years! From such statistics on large population groups, it's safe to say that regular exercise does not shorten life.

Question #3:   Does Exercise Provoke Sudden Cardiac Death?

As we've mentioned several times before, the most recent study attempting to answer this question was published by Dr. Siscovick and his colleagues in the *New England Journal of Medicine* in 1984. On the basis of their data, the authors concluded that the risk of primary cardiac arrest is greater during vigorous exercise than at rest. But at the same time, this increase in risk is greatest among men who are the most sedentary.

Overall, however, habitual exercise is associated with a *decreased* risk for primary cardiac arrest. At our Institute for Aerobics Research, Dr. Larry Gibbons and his colleagues conducted a study, "The Acute Cardiac Risk of Strenuous Exercise," which was reported in a 1980 article in the *Journal of the American Medical Association.* During a sixty-five-month period, 2,935 adults exercised a total of 374,728 hours, including 1,635,763 miles of running and walking. During this time, there were only two cardiac events and *no* deaths.

As of the publication of this book, those numbers have increased to more than 5,000 adults who have walked and run more than 6 million miles. And still, there have been only those two previously reported nonfatal cardiac events.

These data now represent more than thirteen years of follow-up and do not include all the other types of physical activity in which people engage at the Aerobics Center. For example, we have people participating regularly in basketball, racquetball, aerobic dancing, swimming, and other vigorous types of exercise. In light of this evidence, then, the risk of sudden cardiac death during exercise appears to be extremely low—provided basic safety guidelines are followed. These guidelines have been discussed extensively in previous chapters in this book.

Question #4: Does Habitual Exercise Provide Any Immunity Against Infection?

Many regular exercisers, including myself, have noted some protection against infections. This could account for the decreased absenteeism seen in response to industrial fitness programs.

Is there a change in the immune system that can account for this seeming protection?

To help answer this question, Dr. Harvey B. Simon reviewed the immunology of exercise in an article in the November 16, 1984 issue of the *Journal of the American Medical Association*. His conclusions were that exercise does produce a transient increase in white blood cells and in the lymphocytes that are the body's main line of defense against infections. But further studies will be needed before we can conclude absolutely that exercise provides clinically meaningful protection.

Question #5: Does Regular Exercise Cause Cancer or Does it Protect Against Cancer?

Preliminary results of a study released the week of February 10, 1985, produced newspaper headlines such as "Study Indicates Vigorous Exercise May Harm Health." Since that time, inquiries have come to the Cooper Clinic from everywhere. Some people are genuinely concerned; others are more curious than worried. But how much should you be concerned, particularly if you have been exercising for years?

The results of the study referred to above were presented at an international meeting on cancer sponsored by the University of California and the National Foundation for Cancer Research. The study monitored the effect of vigorous exercise on guinea pigs and rats. These animals ran continuously on tiny treadmills for up to two hours daily. In response to such activity, the investigators found that the chemical substance known as free radicals was released. The possibility of free radicals being a cause of cancer is currently a hot subject in the field of cancer research. Yet, the investigators did not find that the exercising experimental animals actually developed cancer. They merely theorized that this was a possibility.

Several things need to be considered regarding this study. First, there is the extent of the exercise. Were these conditioned or deconditioned experimental animals? Regardless, two hours of continuous exercise on a treadmill is fairly demanding for any animal, human or experimental. In this case, exercise might be classified as having more of a straining than training effect. Also, terminology that you will be hearing more about in the future is "eustress" versus "distress." Eustress is normal stress, and when related to exercise, it is not that demanding. Distress is exhaustive exercise that may lead to muscle damage and chronic fatigue. In the case of the experimental animals, I believe it is safe to say they were in a state of distress. Second, conditions might have been right for developing a cancer, yet it was not proven that cancers actually occurred.

But what do we really know about physical activity either causing cancer or protecting us against cancer?

To answer that question, I researched the medical literature and found that epidemiological research does not support a positive exercise-cancer association. To the contrary, being more physically active may actually protect you against cancer, particularly cancer of the colon. Garabrant et al. (*American Journal of Epidemiology* 119:1005–14, 1984) studied the association between occupational activity and cancer in 2,950 male colon cancer patients. Men with sedentary occupations had a colon cancer risk 1.6 times greater than men with high activity occupations. At least two studies, Rusch (*Proceedings of the National Academy of Science U.S.A.* 76:457, 1979) and

Hoffman (*Cancer Research* 22:597, 1962), showed that exercise in animals actually inhibits tumor growth.

Persky et al. (*American Journal of Epidemiology* 114:477–87, 1981) found that a higher resting heart rate was strongly associated with increased colon cancer mortality. These studies strongly indicate that exercise may actually lower colon cancer mortality. Recent studies on Harvard alumni by Paffenbarger are even more impressive (*Journal of the American Medical Association* Vol. 252, No. 4, July 27, 1984). In his study, 16,936 men were followed from 1962 until 1978. Those men expending less than 500 kilocalories per week in physical activity had a cancer death rate of 25.7 per 10,000 man years, as compared to 19.2 for those men expending over 500 kilocalories per week. This was a statistically significant difference. Remember, 500 kilocalories is about what you would use in running a total of five miles in one week.

If there is some protection from cancer offered by exercise, how could this be mediated? One possible answer comes from the work of Dr. Lee S. Berk, Loma Linda University Medical Center, Loma Linda, California. He has been studying the body's defense mechanism against cancer. The immunology against bacterial and viral infections is well known, but less is known about any protection against cancer.

Nonetheless, recent investigators have identified the presence of so-called "natural killers," or NK cells, in the body. Apparently, they are specific against certain types of cancer. They are the body's first line of defense against cancer. Think of these NK cells as bullets that strike and destroy cancer cells in the body, preventing reproduction and ultimately tumor growth. Dr. Berk has now shown that in response to exercise, these NK cells parallel the increase in endorphins. As the endorphin levels increase, so do the NK cells, provided the exercise is in the eustress category. If the exercise is too vigorous or exhaustive (distress), then the NK cells' effectiveness is diminished. In the presence of this detrimental response, the body tries to adapt or condition, and that is why repetitive distress exercise may ultimately become eustress. That is what we call achieving a training effect. Consequently, any detrimental, destructive effect of exercise on NK cells is only transient, provided the exercise becomes regular and consistent. It is the intermittent or sporadic vigorous distress type of exercise that has the potential for long-term harmful effects.

In conclusion, it is impossible at this time to respond more completely to the study reporting increased cancer risk with exercise, since I have seen it only in a newspaper article. I will look forward to the published article and to learning the details of the study. Whether dietary conditions such as excess vitamins or vitamin deficiencies in the presence of vigorous exercise are also cancer-producing, as mentioned in the article, is an unanswered question.

Furthermore, the report states that vigorous exercise accelerates aging. There are many studies showing that exercise retards aging rather than speeds it up. I will continue to question any link between cancer, aging, and regular eustress type of exercise, and I am convinced there is no such data currently in the literature.

Question #6:   Does Regular Exercise Do Anything to Counteract the Effect of Smoking?

Contrary to what many smokers would like to believe, exercise can't counteract the damage being done to your body while you continue to smoke. But what exercise can do is help you kick the habit.

According to one study, smokers who get involved in aerobic exercise become more aware of how smoking has decreased their ability to process oxygen. In short, they find they become winded more easily than their fellow exercisers. This helps create a desire to quit smoking. Vigorous exercise can also help reduce nervous tension, which often leads people to pick up a cigarette.

I have received hundreds of letters from cigarette smokers telling me how they could never break the habit until they started exercising. Regular aerobic activity seems to have given them an overall discipline and self-confidence that they didn't have before.

Question #7: Can Exercise Reduce High Blood Pressure?

People with high blood pressure are prime candidates for a heart attack or a stroke, and the usual treatment has been drugs, weight loss, and a salt-free diet.

But what about exercise? To date, there has been no strong evidence proving that aerobic exercise can reduce blood pressure which is higher than normal. But researchers are coming up with data suggesting that there is a link between exercise and hypertension.

In a study of nearly 17,000 Harvard alumni, Dr. Ralph Paffenbarger has reported that an active lifestyle reduced the risk of coronary heart disease for those with hypertension. Also, there was an interesting twist about the importance of heredity in this study: The physically active alumni who had parents with high blood pressure were at much lower risk for heart disease than the inactive alumni who had hypertensive parents.

Another study, done by Dr. Steven Blair and other researchers from our Institute for Aerobics Research, looked into the association between physical fitness and the development of hypertension in 6,000 healthy men and women without high blood pressure. After following these individuals for almost five years, the researchers found that the risk of developing high blood pressure was considerably higher in those who ranked in the lower fitness categories.

John Duncan, a research associate at the Institute for Aerobics Research, has also been exploring the effects of exercise on people with high blood pressure. In a study lasting sixteen weeks, he focussed on people who had diastolic blood pressures of 90 to 104.

A group of about fifty of these hypertensive people exercised by walking and jogging three times a week for twenty to thirty minutes at a time. A smaller group of fifteen, acting as a "control" against which the others could be measured, did no exercise.

The results were quite encouraging: Seventy percent of the group that exercised lowered their blood pressure to a level below 90. The remaining 30 percent lowered their blood pressure, but not far enough for them to be able to eliminate the use of medication. There were no significant changes that occurred in the nonexercising control group.

In this same study, we also made some discoveries about the physical mechanism through which exercise reduces blood pressure. It seems that aerobic activity reduces the output of noradrenaline, a hormone that can cause high blood pressure by constricting the blood vessels.

Much more work needs to be done before we have a complete understanding of the relationship between exercise and the lowering of high blood pressure. But there's certainly enough evidence at this point for me to say that a regular endurance exercise program may very well help you avoid or control hypertension—and also add years to your life.

Question #8:   Can Exercise Affect the Level of Cholesterol in the Blood?

As you know, cholesterol, the fatty substance found in your cell tissues and bloodstream, has been linked to that great sudden-death threat, arteriosclerosis. So anything that will control the cholesterol in your blood should reduce your chances of heart disease and sudden death. At the same time, you'll increase your chances for a longer life.

Whether exercise lowers total cholesterol, irrespective of changes in diet and body weight, is still being debated. Cross-sectional studies of levels of fitness and selected coronary risk factors showed an inverse relationship between treadmill-determined levels of fitness and serum cholesterol in almost 3,000 men. In other words, those men in the highest categories of fitness had the lowest total cholesterol, and those in the bottom categories of fitness had the highest cholesterols. The differences were significant. (See the *Journal of the American Medical Association,* July 12, 1976, Vol. 236, No. 2.)

In a cross-sectional study of 3,900 adult women reported in 1983 in *Circulation,* no association was found between treadmill-determined levels of fitness and total cholesterol. But there was a strong correlation between fitness on the one hand and the levels of HDL cholesterol and the all-important total cholesterol/HDL ratios on the other.

In addition, Dr. Steven Blair and other researchers reported on a longitudinal study in 1983 in the *American Journal of Epidemiology.* Their investigation showed that among 753 middle-aged men, there was a direct relationship between increased levels of fitness, as determined by treadmill times, and HDL cholesterol. Both the total cholesterol/HDL ratio and the diastolic blood pressure decreased as fitness improved.

To help you understand the full import of these findings, let me take a moment to refresh your memory on some points we discussed in an earlier chapter. The cholesterol that is transported in your blood stream is referred to as total or serum cholesterol. It consists primarily of low density lipoprotein (LDL) and high density lipoprotein (HDL).

In common parlance, LDL is called "bad" cholesterol because it appears that it contributes to the buildup of fatty deposits in the blood vessels. HDL is called "good" cholesterol because it apparently neutralizes the harmful effects of the LDL cholesterol.

A good strategy for developing healthier blood and achieving a longer life is to try to reduce the LDLs in your blood and increase the HDLs. To this end, considerable research has revealed that the levels of the "good" HDL cholesterol can be raised by aerobic exercise. Furthermore, a subcomponent of HDL cholesterol, a substance called HDL-2, is thought to be the basic substance that actually sweeps away the bad cholesterol. This is apparently the key component that goes up with exercise.

Furthermore, numerous studies have shown that active, lean people have a lower LDL count than do those who are inactive and more obese. This is due in part to the lower amount of fat in the fit person's body; in part to the exercise itself; and in part to the better diet of the typical exerciser.

One interesting study along these lines, which was reported in the *Journal of the American Medical Association* in 1984, was done with eleven healthy men and women in their sixties. After a twelve-month exercise training program, their LDL cholesterol levels were lowered, and their HDL cholesterol levels were raised.

This study also found that exercise can increase the body's sensitivity to insulin and glucose. Deterioration of this sensitivity commonly occurs among the aged and may result in diabetes. So, mark up another point for exercise as an important factor in achieving energetic, healthy old age!

But remember: The best way to lower total cholesterol is through changes in diet and weight.

Question #9: Can Exercise Help Me Recover My Health and Increase My Life Span If I've Had a Heart Attack or Bypass Surgery?

Carefully supervised studies on patients recovering from heart attacks and bypass surgery have established that exercise is as important for them as it is for healthy people.

For instance, take the cholesterol levels in those recovering from heart disease. In one British study, forty men from ages twenty-nine to fifty-six who had heart disease were put on a three-week exercise program. The exercise consisted of aerobic activities that raised the heart rate to 80 percent of its maximum level during three twenty-minute periods daily, five times a week. After this routine, the HDL cholesterol levels of all the men who didn't smoke rose significantly. For the men who had continued to smoke, the change in HDLs was negligible.

In a study performed by the Veterans Administration and reported in 1984 in the *New England Journal of Medicine,* eighty-two patients were followed for ten years after bypass surgery. Of 132 grafts shown to be open and working one year after surgery, only fifty were unaffected by arteriosclerosis after the ten-year mark. Among those patients who didn't develop clogged arteries, levels of HDL cholesterol were higher and levels of LDL apoprotein B were lower.

In this investigation no effort was made to correlate physical activity with the presence or absence of new arteriosclerosis or with the levels of HDL cholesterol. But again, we can assume from this data that if exercise does lower LDL levels and increase HDL cholesterol, such activity should be of great benefit to coronary bypass patients.

Also, patients recovering from bypass surgery found that their emotional moods improve after exercise. In fact, according to one researcher, Dr. Albert Oberman of the University of Alabama Medical School, "An improved psyche may be the most striking benefit of a supervised exercise program."

We have frequently found at the Aerobics Center that cardiac rehabilitation patients actually get in better shape *after* bypass surgery than they were in before! As you'll recall, several instances of this sort of thing have already been cited in previous chapters of this book.

So at this point, the evidence is impressive: Exercise—along with a complete rehabilitation program that includes a good, low-fat diet, regular medical checkups, and appropriate changes in lifestyle—can make the "after" condition of the heart patient even better than the "before" state.

In one trial of exercise training in randomly selected patients with coronary heart disease, Dr. Victor Froelicher and other researchers showed that after one year of supervised exercise, there were significant differences between the exercise and control groups. These investigators reported in a 1984 article in the *Journal of the American Medical Association* that the exercise group showed modest but encouraging signs of improvement: They increased their aerobic capacity, thallium ischemia scores, and ventricular function.

As for whether exercise increases the heart patient's life span, that's an issue that hasn't been completely settled. Yet support for this conclusion is growing throughout the medical literature.

For example, Dr. G. S. May and his associates reviewed the results of exercise training among patients who had suffered heart attacks in a 1982 article in the journal *Progressive Cardiovascular Disease*. They examined six studies of 2,752 patients that used random assignment to exercise or control groups. None of the studies individually demonstrated a significant effect of exercise.

But when the results were *pooled,* there was a 19 percent reduction in total mortality in the exercise group! Also, there was *no* increase in deaths from exercise training, even in those patients with known coronary heart disease. The benefits of exercise appeared to have far outweighed any risks. I firmly believe that future studies will show even more dramatically that exercise does increase the life expectancy of cardiac patients.

But whether you're a heart patient or not, if you hope to increase your life span, it's necessary to return to the basic guidelines that we began with in this chapter. In short, you must immediately incorporate into your daily existence those four basic Longevity Habits—medical exams with stress tests; proper weight, maintained with a low-fat, high-fiber diet; regular endurance exercise; and an avoidance of tobacco.

And that means following *all* of these practices, without exception. Only then can you hope to maximize your chances of staying one step ahead of such specters as heart disease and sudden death.

CHAPTER TEN

BEYOND THE JIM FIXX SYNDROME: THE FUTURE OF THE EXERCISE BOOM

Fads come and go swiftly in America and many other countries, as manufacturers well know. The public taste is often unpredictable, despite all the poll-taking and marketing research we do.

So, what about the aerobic exercise boom? Will it, in the end, prove to be just another fleeting fancy? Or are we involved in something that seems destined to stay with us and perhaps permanently change our way of life?

Certainly, until the death of Jim Fixx, there were many solid signs that endurance exercise would be a part of our lives for the foreseeable future. Enthusiasm bordering on euphoria and even religious ecstasy sometimes accompanied exercise: We heard clamors of, "The more, the better!" We've seen television commercials, magazine ads, and books by celebrities extolling the Body Beautiful as the ultimate goal in life.

Then Jim Fixx collapsed on that lonely rural road in northern Vermont, and the cheering began to fade away. If such a magnificent symbol of fitness and health could die during a routine run, what about the rest of us?

191

A few strenuous opponents of aerobic exercise, some from re-spected corners of the medical community, emerged at this point and went on the attack. They had been cautious before because they had no compelling cause or symbol to embrace. But now, they had Jim Fixx. Using his tragedy as their rallying cry, they relied heavily on fear in their efforts to stem the tide of the exercise movement, and perhaps even reverse it.

As a follow-up to Jim Fixx's death, some exercise critics were saying that it's possible to be aerobically fit and still not be healthy. I'm sure that if Jim Fixx had been evaluated on a treadmill, he would have scored in the excellent or superior category for his sex and age. But was he really healthy?

The answer is no, he wasn't healthy. Nor would I have classified him as such if, as I expect, his treadmill stress ECG had been grossly abnormal. So there's a difference between physical fitness and health, and the treadmill stress ECG helps us to make that distinction. If a patient ranks in the good or a higher physical fitness category and his stress ECG is normal, I would say that, from the standpoint of the cardiovascular system, he is *both* fit and healthy.

But now, the potential for this brand of panic and negative think-ing seems to have passed. Instead, after all the questioning and soul-searching about the meaning of Jim's death, we appear to be moving into a more mature phase of the exercise movement. We seem to have entered an era that will allow us to approach aerobic activity as an important tool to combat heart disease and sudden death, but not a panacea.

In short, we're moving beyond a belief in the myths about exer-cise that comprise the Jim Fixx Syndrome. We no longer believe that exercise eliminates the need for regular physical exams . . . that the more you exercise, the more protection you'll get from heart disease . . . that running a marathon virtually ensures that you're protected from a heart attack . . . or that endurance exercise can completely overcome the negative effects of a bad diet or a family history of heart trouble.

Myths like these could indeed threaten the exercise boom, mostly because they are so patently false. But against these misconceptions, there are important current trends, based on the incontrovertible facts about the value of exercise, which make the future of the move-ment firm and secure.

What are those trends? I've identified at least four, and I believe they'll continue to grow stronger in the years ahead.

Trend #1:   Public Opinion

In 1961, the Gallup Poll first asked the question, "Aside from any work you do at home or at a job, do you do anything regularly—that is, on a daily basis—that helps you keep physically fit?" At that time, only 24 percent of the population responded "yes." In 1984, however, twenty-three years later, 59 percent, over half of the population, replied that they exercised on a regular basis.

The more than doubling of regular exercisers in a period of slightly more than two decades indicates to me that physical fitness has become more than just a passing interest for Americans. Many of these fitness enthusiasts are joggers: About one in seven adults and more than half of the teenagers surveyed said they engage in this activity. Significantly, a typical run for adults was 2.3 miles, and for teenagers was 2.6 miles. Those figures reflect distances being run by people who take endurance exercise seriously. Moreover, in light of the number of youngsters who are running, the numbers in the survey bode well for the future of aerobic activity. Finally, in an equally impressive development, the number of participants in aerobic dancing programs is now estimated to exceed 18 million.

Trend #2:   The Insurance Companies

Even though a huge amount of their own money is on the line in the form of premiums and payouts for benefits, the insurance industry has been much less conservative than the medical profession in recognizing the benefits of exercise.

Allstate Life Insurance Company, a member of the Sears Financial Network, is offering up to a 35 percent discount for those subscribers who exercise regularly. Other insurance companies are offering discounts as high as 50 percent to nonsmokers who are also involved in physical fitness programs. Most of these insurance organizations require a minimum of thirty minutes of cardiovascular exercise (such as running or swimming) at least three times a week in order to qualify for the discount.

And that's not all. The Executive Life Insurance Company of Beverly Hills, California, offers what they have termed a "Sweatshirt Rate" for clients who agree to submit to yearly physicals.

Worth Wilson of Occidental Life Insurance Company summed it up boldly in *USA Today* by saying, "If you're going to live longer, you should get a break on your insurance costs."

Trend #3:   Big Corporations

Companies have been hit hard by the ever-increasing rates of health insurance, and so they have begun to look around for ways to reduce their health insurance premiums.

An article in a 1983 issue of the *Journal of the American Medical Association* reported that several major companies have already spent millions to develop fitness and other health plans for their employees. These companies include Kimberly Clark, Johnson & Johnson, Sentry Insurance, Campbell's Soup Company, Pepsico, and Holiday Inns.

Dr. Donald W. Bowne and his associates at the Prudential Insurance Company recently published an impressive study that documents how disability and health care costs can be reduced through an industrial fitness program. As related in a 1984 article in the *Journal of Occupational Medicine,* these researchers studied 1,389 employees of their company over a five-year period. The participants showed a 45.7 percent reduction in major medical costs, rather than the expected inflationary increase.

There was also a reduction of 20.1 percent in the average number of disability days and a 31.7 percent reduction in direct disability dollar costs in the year after the study. Those participating were well-educated and most held sedentary, white-collar jobs. Their involvement was voluntary and without any financial incentives. In dollars-and-cents terms, the average combined savings per participant were $353.38, and the average operational cost was $120.60. These results strongly suggest that work-site wellness programs can make a substantial contribution to the reduction of health care and disability costs. Clearly, there is a reason corporations are betting big money on the health benefits from a continuing exercise boom.

Trend #4: Government Policies

The interest in physical fitness has caught the imagination of governments around the world. I see this trend firsthand as I meet with government leaders in Europe, South America, and the Far East. I'm always especially impressed when I travel to Brazil for a regular government-sponsored run through the streets of Rio. And the word about exercise is clearly still spreading.

In March 1984, Indonesia announced that it had launched a nationwide get-fit program. The program was designed to encourage Indonesians to work out at least once a week. And one month later, sports training was scheduled to become compulsory for the country's 5 million civil servants. The evidence suggests strongly that even more nations will hop on the exercise bandwagon in the future.

In the United States, many national fitness programs have been launched and goals for the future set in recent years. For example, the U.S. Department of Health and Human Services has recently established eleven goals for exercise that they expect to see achieved by 1990. These include such sweeping reforms as:

- getting more than 90 percent of youngsters aged ten to seventeen participating regularly in cardiovascular fitness programs;
- getting more than 60 percent of adults from age eighteen to sixty-five involved in vigorous physical exercise; and
- getting 50 percent of adults sixty-five and over involved in aerobic activities like walking and swimming.

What all this adds up to is a worldwide movement toward physical fitness that simply can't be denied. We've moved beyond fantasy to the reality that cardiovascular fitness can indeed reduce the risks of killer diseases and enhance the prospects for a longer, more energetic life.

And the tragedy of Jim Fixx has done as much if not more than any other single event to help us focus our attention on the proper role that exercise should play in a complete preventive health program. Now, because of our agonizing analyses of why he died and what that means to each of us personally, we are in a better position to select the safest exercise programs. We can see more clearly how exercise can reduce the risk of heart disease and sudden death.

So finally, as you get involved in your own personal exercise program, *burn* these basic guidelines into your mind, so that they become as much second-nature to you as the physical activity itself:

- Obtain medical clearance, including treadmill stress testing on a regular basis, adjusted to age and coronary risk factors.
- Slowly progress into any vigorous exercise program.
- Adequately warm up to avoid both musculo-skeletal and cardiovascular problems.
- Exercise aerobically with enough duration, intensity, and frequency to condition the cardiovascular system properly.
- Be aware of the possibility of overuse of the body, which may be associated with chronic musculo-skeletal or cardiac problems.
- Avoid sudden increases in physical activity, such as doubling the weekly mileage.
- Cool down properly following vigorous aerobic activity to avoid "post-exercise peril."
- Seek medical attention anytime there are persistent or abnormal symptoms.

If you keep these principles in mind and begin to live by them, you should be able to run, swim, ski, dance, cycle, or pursue any exercise with greater confidence—and without fear!

APPENDIX

Recommendations for the Frequency of Exercise Testing Under the Cooper Protocol

1. Maximal rather than submaximal testing should be used whenever possible. A maximal exercise test has a greater chance of revealing evidence of unsuspected coronary disease and is a much more reliable estimate of maximal oxygen consumption.

2. The treadmill time and incline guidelines of the Balke Protocol should be used. This protocol has been employed in all previous research at the Aerobics Center and has proven to be a safe procedure. The longer treadmill times required under the Balke Protocol also make it easier to quantify and compare levels of fitness.

3. Specific recommendations for frequency of exercise testing:

A. *Apparently Healthy Individuals:*
Apparently healthy individuals below age forty can generally start exercising without exercise testing, with two important qualifications: 1) The exercise must begin and proceed gradually, and 2) the individual must watch for the occurrence of new signs or symptoms. At age forty or above, it is desirable for these individuals to have a maximal exercise test prior to undertaking

an exercise program. Thereafter, exercise testing should be done at least every three years.

B. Individuals at Higher Risk:

These individuals at higher risk have at least one major coronary risk factor, among those listed below:

1. Cigarette smoking
2. Elevated total cholesterol/high density lipoprotein (HDL) cholesterol ratio (above 5.0 for males or 4.5 for females)
3. High blood pressure (greater than 145/95)
4. Abnormal resting ECG
5. Diabetes mellitus
6. Family history of coronary disease at age fifty or before

Also, higher-risk individuals include those with symptoms suggestive of cardiopulmonary or metabolic disease.

For those with risk factors but no symptoms, an exercise test is not necessary below age thirty-five if the exercise is undertaken gradually, with appropriate progression. But persons with symptoms suggestive of heart, lung, or metabolic disease should have a supervised maximum exercise test prior to beginning a vigorous exercise program at any age. Following exercise testing, a decision can be made as to whether or not the symptoms appear to be related to underlying disease. After initial testing, individuals in this higher-risk category should have exercise testing every two years.

C. Patients with Disease:

Individuals with known cardiovascular, pulmonary, or metabolic disease should have an exercise test prior to beginning vigorous exercise at any age. These individuals or any person with an abnormal exercise test should have repeat exercise testing annually.

4. In order to classify individuals into one of these three categories it is necessary for them to fill out a brief medical questionnaire that asks about symptoms, cigarette usage, and family history. It is also necessary to measure the total cholesterol to HDL ratio, blood pressure, and blood sugar. In addition, they must have a resting ECG.

5. It is advisable for healthy adults to have such a screening check of major risk factors at least every five years until age thirty-five, and at least every three years thereafter.

Basic Rules for Safe and Sensitive Maximal-Performance Treadmill Stress Testing

1. Proper selection of patients. (Know the conditions for which stress testing is contraindicated.)

2. Use of appropriate treadmill testing techniques (e.g., Balke, Bruce, or a modified test).

3. Multilead monitoring (at least seven electrodes on the chest monitoring nine of the twelve standard ECG leads).

4. Maximal performance (exceeding 85 percent of PMHR, using either 220 minus age for women and unfit men or 205 minus one-half age for conditioned men).

5. Properly trained physicians and technicians, knowledgeable in interpreting an electrocardiogram and in handling resuscitation equipment.

Absolute Contraindications to Stress Testing or Exercise Participation

1. Unstable or crescendo angina.

2. Acute myocardial infarction (less than two weeks post-MI).

3. Acute pulmonary embolism or infarction.

4. Tight aortic stenosis or any severe valvular disease.

5. Uncontrolled ventricular or atrial ectopy or arrhythmia.

6. High degrees of heart block (i.e., third-degree atrioventricular block).

7. Untreated atrial fibrillation.

8. Acute or severe congestive heart failure.

9. Decompensated cor pulmonale.

10. Uncontrolled severe hypertension ($> 220/110$) or hypotension ($< 80/—$).

11. Uncontrolled diabetes mellitus.

12. Acute myocarditis, pericarditis, or rheumatic fever; subacute bacterial endocarditis.

13. Uncontrolled systemic disease (i.e., thyroid, hepatic, renal, central nervous system, or malignancy).

14. Suspected or known dissecting aneurysm.

15. Current systemic infection.

16. Psychotic or otherwise mentally unstable or uncooperative patient.

17. Severe anemia or debilitated patients with chronic disease.

18. Acute thrombophlebitis.

19. Fixed-rate pacemakers.

20. Severe physical handicaps (e.g., amputee, severe arthritis, or deformity).

From the Cooper Clinic Protocol and *Exercise Electrocardiography, Practical Approach,* Second Edition, by Edward K. Chung, M.D. Baltimore: Williams & Williams, 1983.

Indications for Stopping a Treadmill Stress Test

1. Failure of monitoring system.

2. Progressive angina (increasing angina is always an indication to stop the test, regardless of any ECG abnormality).

3. Two millimeters horizontal or down-sloping S-T depression or elevation.

4. Sustained supraventricular tachyarrhythmias.

5. Ventricular tachycardia or fibrillation, including three or more grouped premature ventricular contractions.

6. Any significant drop in systolic blood pressure (> 10 mmHg) or heart rate (> 5 beats/min.).

7. Lightheadedness, confusion, cyanosis, pallor, nausea, or ataxia (lack of coordination).

8. The subject wants to stop!

9. Excessive blood pressure ($> 240/120$).

10. Acute myocardial infarction.

Aerobics Center Treadmill
Stress Test Records

Male Name/Home	Time	Age	*Female* Name/Home	Time
Blake Boyd, Texas	32:10	Under 20	Terrie Brown, Texas	29:35
Kyle Heffner, Texas	37:07	20–24	Ann Bond, Texas	30:00
Mark Hunter, Texas	35:00	25–29	Deborah Strehle, Texas	32:30
Norbert Sanders, New York	36:00	30–34	Eleonora Mendonca, Brazil	32:10
Jim Ryun, Kansas	36:16	35–39	Sharon O'Connor, Colorado	33:00
Brian Bolton, Texas	34:30	40–44	Mary Jones, Texas	29:32
Paul Vernon, Texas	34:34	45–49	Anne Zink, Iowa	28:04
Allen Thomson, New Zealand	32:32	50–54	Gloria McLeod, Texas	25:35
Arno Jensen, Texas	30:35	55–59	Gloria McLeod, Texas	24:42
Richard Parkinson, California	30:32	60–64	Marion Read, Wisconsin	21:00
George Sheehan, New Jersey	30:02	65–69	Constance Hughes, Alabama	21:05
Ralph Osborn, Texas	27:35	70–74	Polly Clarke, Colorado	22:00
Johnny Kelly, Massachusetts	25:00	75–79		
John Clark, Colorado	25:00			
Arlitt Allsup, Texas	12:00	80–over	Helen Bailey, California	7:30

January 23, 1985

Relative Contraindications to Stress Testing or Exercise Participation

Note: Individuals having one or more of these medical conditions should not be stress tested unless the procedure is done under close medical supervision, nor should they be permitted to enter any exercise program unless it is professionally supervised. This material is taken from the Cooper Clinic Protocol and from *Exercise Electrocardiography, Practical Approach,* Second Edition, by Edward K. Chung, M.D. Baltimore: Williams & Williams, 1983.

1. Clinically significant noncardiac medical problems.

2. Anemia (less than 10 gms Hgb) but under treatment; hemorrhagic diseases such as hemophilia.

3. Moderate to severe hypertension ($> 180/100$).

4. Pulmonary hypertension due to chronic obstructive pulmonary disease.

5. Fractures, dislocations, tendon or cartilaginous injuries affecting locomotion, during the period of injury.

6. Severe arthritic conditions.

7. Convulsive disorders not controlled by medication.

8. History of intracranial bleeding within the past six months.

9. Controlled systemic diseases, such as renal, hepatic, central nervous system, or malignancy.

10. History of recent or active gastrointestinal bleeding.

11. History of recent surgery until completely ambulatory (usually six weeks before full program participation is permitted).

12. Any severe heart disease other than those given under Absolute Contraindications (see list in Appendix).

13. Moderate to severe pulmonary insufficiency.

Common Causes for False-Negative Treadmill Stress Tests

Note: This section refers to false negatives for obstructive coronary artery disease.

1. Drugs (nitroglycerin, Isordil, and other anti-anginal drugs; phenothiazines, procainamide).

2. Myocardial and coronary artery abnormalities (old myocardial infarction, single-vessel coronary artery disease, coronary artery obstruction less than 60 percent of the lumen).

3. Submaximal test (early cessation of test at less than 85 percent predicted maximum heart rate, due to anxiety, deconditioning, lack of motivation).

4. Inadequate lead system (not monitoring at least nine of the twelve standard ECG leads before, during, and after the test).

5. Miscellaneous (LAD, left anterior hemiblock).

6. Failure to use other available information (i.e., fall in heart rate or systolic BP, chest pain).

Common Causes for False-Positive Treadmill Stress Tests

Note: This section refers to false positives for obstructive coronary artery disease.

1. Drugs (digitalis, diuretics, beta-blockers, Quinidine, sedatives, antidepressant drugs, estrogen).

2. Hypertension ($> 240/120$).

3. Electrolyte deficiency (hypokalemia or low potassium is the most common cause).

4. T-wave lability (postural or hyperventilation changes) or non-specific ST-T wave changes.

5. Valvular (mitral valve prolapse, aortic stenosis).

6. Preexisting conduction defects (left bundle branch block, right bundle branch block, WPW syndrome).

7. Myocardial abnormalities (left ventricular hypertrophy, right ventricular hypertrophy, coronary artery bridging, asymmetric septal hypertrophy, idiopathic hypertrophic subaortic stenosis, hypertrophic cardiomyopathy, old myocardial infarction, myocarditis, rheumatic heart disease, hypertensive heart disease).

8. Miscellaneous (food intake, pectus excavation, sudden intense exercise).

Comments: Even though the above may cause false-positive tests for obstructive coronary artery disease, they are not necessarily false positive from the standpoint of heart disease. When a classic ischemic S-T segment is seen on a stress ECG, usually some pathology can be found to explain it.

Canadian Physical Activity Readiness Questionnaire

If any of the following questions are answered yes, physical activity might be inappropriate and medical advice should be sought regarding the type and intensity of exercise permissible.

_____ Has your doctor ever said you have heart trouble?

_____ Do you frequently suffer from pains in your heart or chest?

_____ Do you often feel faint or have episodes of severe dizziness?

_____ Has a doctor ever said your blood pressure was too high?

_____ Has a doctor ever told you that you have a bone or joint problem such as arthritis that has been aggravated by exercise or might be made worse with exercise?

_____ Is there a good physical reason not mentioned above why you should not follow an activity program, even if you wanted to?

_____ Are you over age 69 and not accustomed to vigorous exercise?

Reference: Par-Q Validation Report, British Columbia Department of Health, June 1975 (modified version).

Exercise ECG Evaluations—Cooper Clinic

Impressions:

☐ Normal Exercise Tolerance Test

☐ Inconclusive Test

    ☐ Submaximal (less than 85% predicted maximum heart rate)

    ☐ Systems failure

    ☐ Drug effect (name of drug) _____

    ☐ Other (specify) _____

☐ Equivocal Exercise Tolerance Test

    ☐ S-T segment depression or elevation 0.5 mm to $<$ 1 mm in amplitude $\geq$ .08 sec.

    ☐ PVC's 10% or more ($>$ 10/100) in any minute of test

    ☐ Supraventricular tachycardia

    ☐ Excessive hypertension ($>$ 240/120)

    ☐ T-wave changes (not postural or with hyperventilation)

    ☐ Other (specify) _____

☐ Abnormal Exercise Tolerance Test

    ☐ Horizontal or down-sloping S-T segment depression, $\geq$ 1 mm $\geq$ .08 sec.

	Rest	*Submax.*	*Max.*	*Recovery*
_____ I	N	N	Abn°	N
_____ II	N	Abn	N	N
_____ III	N	N	N	Abn
_____ IV	N	N	Abn	Abn
_____ V	N	Abn	Abn	Abn
_____ VI	Abn	Abn°°	—	Abn

° Abnormal only during final 1–2 minutes of true maximal performance
°° Stopped at low heart rate due to very abnormal ECG ($>$ 2 mm S-T↓)

☐ Horizontal or up-sloping S-T segment elevation (≥ 1 mm)

☐ Typical angina or chest pain

☐ Hypotension in the presence of an increasing workload

☐ Inappropriate bradycardia (a decreasing heart rate in the presence of an increasing workload)

☐ Exercise-induced $2°$ or $3°$ heart block

☐ R or T PVC's

☐ Unifocal PVC's greater than 20% in any minute of test

☐ Couplets of PVC's with known coronary artery disease or S-T depression ≥ 1 mm $\geq .08$ sec.

☐ Ventricular tachycardia ($>$ three PVC's together)

☐ LBB _____ or RBBB _____ (induced)

☐ Multifocal PVC's

☐ Inverted U waves

☐ Other (specify) _____

Comments:

- If S-T↓ ≥ 2 mm + freq. PVC's, or multifocal PVC's, or grouped PVC's, or marked bradycardia, this is usually diagnostic of advanced multi-vessel coronary artery disease.
- If S-T↓ ≥ 2 mm lasting .08 sec., this is much more ominous in the presence of ventricular ectopy.
- If S-T↓ ≥ 2 mm lasting .08 sec. occurs at low heart rates, this indicates severe coronary artery disease.
- If S-T is down-sloping in recovery only, this is more likely a false positive.
- If S-T is depressed and horizontal in recovery only, this is more likely a true positive.

Predicted Maximum Heart Rates in Men, According to Physical Fitness Categories

Age	Below Average	Average	Above Average, Good, Excellent, Superior	Age	Below Average	Average	Above Average, Good, Excellent, Superior
20	201	201	196	45	174	183	183
21	199	200	196	46	173	182	183
22	198	199	195	47	172	181	182
23	197	198	195	48	171	181	182
24	196	198	194	49	170	180	181
25	195	197	194	50	168	179	180
26	194	196	193	51	167	179	180
27	193	196	193	52	166	178	179
28	192	195	192	53	165	177	179
29	191	193	192	54	164	176	178
30	190	193	191	55	163	176	178
31	189	193	191	56	162	175	177
32	188	192	190	57	161	174	177
33	187	191	189	58	160	174	176
34	186	191	189	59	159	173	176
35	184	190	188	60	158	172	175
36	183	189	188	61	157	172	175
37	182	189	187	62	156	171	174
38	181	188	187	63	155	170	174
39	180	187	186	64	154	169	173
40	180	186	185	65	152	169	173
41	178	186	185	66	151	168	172
42	177	185	185	67	150	167	171
43	176	184	184	68	149	167	171
44	175	184	184	69	148	166	170
				70	147	165	170

Observed Maximal Heart Rates in Women, According to Physical Fitness Categories

Age	Below Average	Average	Above Average
18–24	191	191	191
25–29	187	189	188
30–34	182	184	185
35–39	181	184	185
40–44	175	180	182
45–49	171	175	178
50–54	167	170	176
55–59	162	166	172
60–64	160	161	166
65–75	146	153	158

From *Physiological Response to Maximal Graded Exercise Testing in Apparently Healthy White Women Aged Eighteen to Seventy-five Years.* Blair et al., *Journal of Cardiac Rehabilitation,* Vol. 4, No. 11, November 1984.

Definition of Fitness Categories for Males

	Age Group (years)				
FITNESS CATEGORY	<30	30–39	40–49	50–59	60 +
☐ VERY POOR	<14:59	<13:09	<11:59	<9:59	<6:59
☐ POOR	15:00–17:29	13:10–15:59	12:00–14:14	10:00–12:06	7:00– 9:99
☐ FAIR	17:30–20:59	16:00–19:59	14:15–17:59	12:07–15:39	10:00–13:21
☐ GOOD	21:00–23:59	20:00–22:59	18:00–20:59	15:40–18:59	13:22–16:59
☐ EXCELLENT	24:00–26:59	23:00–25:59	21:00–24:29	19:00–22:14	17:00–20:55
☐ SUPERIOR	27:00 +	26:00 +	24:30 +	22:15 +	20:56 +

Based on the Cooper Clinic modified Balke treadmill protocol: 3.3 mph (90m/min), 0% for 1st min, 2% for 2nd min, + 1% for each additional min. to 25%, then + .2 mph until exhaustion.

Definition of Fitness Categories for Females

	Age Group (years)				
FITNESS CATEGORY	<30	30–39	40–49	50–59	60 +
☐ VERY POOR	<9:59	<8:59	<7:19	<5:59	<4:59
☐ POOR	10:00–12:16	9:00–11:08	7:20– 9:59	6:00– 7:42	5:00– 6:15
☐ FAIR	12:17–15:29	11:09–14:09	10:00–12:29	7:43–10:13	6:16– 8:59
☐ GOOD	15:30–18:59	14:10–17:29	12:30–15:34	10:14–12:52	9:00–11:59
☐ EXCELLENT	19:00–21:59	17:30–19:59	15:35–17:59	12:53–15:06	12:00–15:33
☐ SUPERIOR	22:00 +	20:00 +	18:00 +	15:07 +	15:34 +

Based on the Cooper Clinic modified Balke treadmill protocol: 3.3 mph (90m/min), 0% for 1st min, 2% for 2nd min, + 1% for each additional min. to 25%, then + .2 mph until exhaustion.

Coronary Risk Factor Charts

The following coronary risk factor charts are completely new and represent data obtained from 27,168 men and women evaluated at the Cooper Clinic (first visit data only). They have been formulated in view of the latest research showing those things in your life that are most likely to cause heart trouble.

To use these charts, first choose the one that correlates with your age and sex. Next, go over the chart with your physician and fill in the blanks in conjunction with your medical examination. You can find the number of points to be awarded each risk factor by looking at the numbers on the left side of each column. You should add up the points you've received for each factor and see where that places you in the Total Coronary Risk box in the lower right-hand corner of each page. At the time of your next examination, you can compare coronary risk points by entering both the current and previous totals.

It is recommended that you try to achieve the fifty-fifth percentile ranking or higher in each of the seven coronary risk factors listed across the top of the page. Overall, try to earn the minimum number of points so that you can be in the lowest overall coronary risk.

A sample coronary risk factor chart is below. Please see the preceding page for an explanation of the charts.

COOPER CLINIC/ Dallas, Texas   *SAMPLE*   **Coronary Risk Profile**

NAME: *JOHN DOE*   **Males: *40-49 Years of Age**

PERCENTILE RANKINGS	BALKE TREADMILL TIME (min.)	TOTAL CHOLESTEROL/ HDL RATIO	TRIGLYCERIDE (mg. %)	GLUCOSE (mg. %)	% BODY FAT	RESTING BLOOD PRESSURE SYSTOLIC (mm HG)	DIASTOLIC (mm HG)
YOUR VALUES	13:50 [4]	4.3 [0]	112 [0]	91 [0]	30.7 [3]	116 [0]	80 [0]
99	28:00	2.6	38.0	77.0	6.6	94.0	60.0
97	25:45	2.9	47.0	81.0	9.9	100.0	65.0
95	24:30	3.1	53.0	84.0	11.4	100.0	68.0
90	23:00	3.4	63.0	87.0	13.6	106.0	70.0
85	21:00	3.6	70.0	89.0	15.1	110.0	72.0
80	20:10	3.8	77.0	91.0	16.3	110.0	74.0
75	20:00	4.1	84.0	92.0	17.3	112.0	76.0
70	18:32	4.2	90.0	94.0	18.1	114.0	78.0
65	18:00	4.4	97.0	95.0	18.8	116.0	78.0
60	17:15	4.6	104.0	97.0	19.6	118.0	80.0
55	17:00	4.8	111.0	98.0	20.3	120.0	80.0
50	16:00	5.0	119.0	99.0	21.1	120.0	80.0
45	15:30	5.2	128.0	100.0	21.8	120.0	80.0
40	15:00	5.4	138.0	102.0	22.5	122.0	82.0
35	14:15	5.7	149.0	104.0	23.3	124.0	84.0
30	13:57	5.9	162.0	105.0	24.1	128.0	86.0
25	13:00	6.2	177.0	107.0	25.0	130.0	88.0
20	12:30	6.5	199.0	109.0	26.1	130.0	90.0
15	12:00	6.9	226.0	111.0	27.3	135.0	90.0
10	10:59	7.5	263.0	115.0	28.9	140.0	94.0
5	9:13	8.4	360.0	120.0	31.5	146.0	100.0
3	8:00	9.0	420.1	125.0	33.4	150.0	102.0
1	6:21	10.6	656.1	147.1	37.4	160.0	110.0
N	6837	3073	6196	6192	5724	6939	6939

PERSONAL HISTORY OF HEART ATTACK OR BYPASS
- 0 ☑ NONE
- 2 ☐ OVER 5 YEARS AGO
- 4 ☐ 2 - 5 YEARS AGO
- 5 ☐ 1 - < 2 YEARS AGO
- 8 ☐ 0 - < 1 YEAR AGO   [0]

FAMILY HISTORY OF CORONARY HEART DISEASE
- 0 ☑ NONE OR OVER 65
- 2 ☐ YES, AGE 50-65
- 4 ☐ YES, UNDER AGE 50   [0]

KNOWN CORONARY HEART DISEASE W/O HEART ATTACK OR BYPASS
- 0 ☑ NONE
- 2 ☐ OVER 5 YEARS AGO
- 4 ☐ 2 - 5 YEARS AGO
- 5 ☐ 1 - < 2 YEARS AGO
- 6 ☐ 0 - < 1 YEAR AGO   [0]

SMOKING HABITS
- 0 ☑ NONE
- 0 ☐ PAST 1 YEAR OR MORE
- 1 ☐ PAST ONLY LESS THAN 1 YEAR
- 1 ☐ PIPE/CIGAR
- 2 ☐ 1 - 10 DAILY
- 3 ☐ 11 - 20 DAILY
- 4 ☐ 21 - 30 DAILY
- 5 ☐ 31 - 40 DAILY
- 6 ☐ MORE THAN 40 DAILY   [0]

TENSION - ANXIETY
- 0 ☐ NO TENSION, VERY RELAXED
- 0 ☐ SLIGHT TENSION
- 1 ☑ MODERATE TENSION
- 2 ☐ HIGH TENSION
- 3 ☐ VERY TENSE, "HIGH STRUNG"   [1]
- 3 ☐ DIABETES   [0]

Data based on first visit only
© Institute for Aerobics Research - 1985

AGE FACTOR
- 0 ☐ UNDER 30 YEARS OF AGE
- 1 ☐ 30 - 39 YEARS OF AGE
- 2 ☑ 40 - 49 YEARS OF AGE
- 3 ☐ 50 - 59 YEARS OF AGE
- 4 ☐ 60 + YEARS OF AGE   [2]

RESTING ECG		EXERCISE ECG	
0 ☑	NORMAL	0 ☑	
1 ☐	EQUIVOCAL	4 ☐	
3 ☐	ABNORMAL	8 ☐	
			[0]

TOTAL CORONARY RISK
- ☐ VERY LOW   (0- 4)
- ☑ LOW   (5-12)
- ☐ MODERATE   (13-21)
- ☐ HIGH   (22-31)
- ☐ VERY HIGH   (32 +)   ——— [10]

PREVIOUS TOTAL   - - - [13]

| NAME: | | | | | | **Males: * < 30 Years of Age** | |

PERCENTILE RANKINGS	BALKE TREADMILL TIME (min.)	TOTAL CHOLESTEROL/ HDL RATIO	TRIGLYCERIDE (mg. %)	GLUCOSE (mg. %)	% BODY FAT	RESTING BLOOD PRESSURE SYSTOLIC (mm HG)	DIASTOLIC (mm HG)
YOUR VALUES							
99	30:20	2.3	31.0	73.0	2.4	92.0	58.0
97	28:22	2.5	39.0	78.0	4.2	98.0	60.0
95	27:00	2.7	44.5	80.0	5.2	100.0	62.0
90	25:11	2.9	50.0	84.0	7.1	104.0	66.0
85	24:00	3.1	55.0	86.0	8.3	108.0	68.0
80	23:00	3.2	60.0	88.0	9.4	110.0	70.0
75	22:10	3.4	64.0	89.0	10.6	112.0	70.0
70	22:00	3.5	69.0	90.0	11.8	114.0	72.0
65	21:00	3.7	74.0	91.0	12.9	116.0	74.0
60	20:15	3.8	79.0	93.0	14.1	118.0	75.0
55	20:00	4.0	84.0	94.0	15.0	120.0	76.0
50	19:03	4.1	89.0	95.0	15.9	120.0	78.0
45	19:00	4.2	95.0	96.0	16.8	120.0	80.0
40	18:00	4.4	102.0	97.0	17.4	122.0	80.0
35	17:30	4.5	111.0	98.0	18.3	124.0	80.0
30	17:00	4.7	122.0	100.0	19.5	126.0	80.0
25	16:00	4.9	131.0	101.0	20.7	128.0	82.0
20	15:20	5.2	145.0	103.0	22.4	130.0	84.0
15	15:00	5.6	168.0	105.0	23.9	132.0	86.4
10	13:30	6.0	190.0	108.0	25.9	138.0	90.0
5	11:30	6.9	245.5	112.0	29.1	142.0	92.0
3	10:06	7.3	289.3	115.0	31.0	146.0	96.0
1	8:23	8.7	420.4	121.1	36.4	155.0	100.0
N	1675	763	1389	1392	1342	1703	1703

PERSONAL HISTORY OF HEART ATTACK OR BYPASS
0 ☐ NONE
2 ☐ OVER 5 YEARS AGO
4 ☐ 2 - 5 YEARS AGO
5 ☐ 1 - 2 YEARS AGO
8 ☐ 0 - 1 YEAR AGO

FAMILY HISTORY OF CORONARY HEART DISEASE
0 ☐ NONE OR OVER 65
2 ☐ YES, AGE 50-65
4 ☐ YES, UNDER AGE 50

KNOWN CORONARY HEART DISEASE W/O HEART ATTACK OR BYPASS
0 ☐ NONE
2 ☐ OVER 5 YEARS AGO
4 ☐ 2 - 5 YEARS AGO
5 ☐ 1 - < 2 YEARS AGO
6 ☐ 0 - < 1 YEAR AGO

SMOKING HABITS
0 ☐ NONE
0 ☐ PAST 1 YEAR OR MORE
1 ☐ PAST ONLY LESS THAN 1 YEAR
1 ☐ PIPE/CIGAR
2 ☐ 1 - 10 DAILY
3 ☐ 11 - 20 DAILY
4 ☐ 21 - 30 DAILY
5 ☐ 31 - 40 DAILY
6 ☐ MORE THAN 40 DAILY

TENSION - ANXIETY
0 ☐ NO TENSION, VERY RELAXED
0 ☐ SLIGHT TENSION
1 ☐ MODERATE TENSION
2 ☐ HIGH TENSION
3 ☐ VERY TENSE, "HIGH STRUNG"

3 ☐ DIABETES

*Data based on first visit only
© Institute for Aerobics Research - 1985

AGE FACTOR
0 ☐ UNDER 30 YEARS OF AGE
1 ☐ 30 - 39 YEARS OF AGE
2 ☐ 40 - 49 YEARS OF AGE
3 ☐ 50 - 59 YEARS OF AGE
4 ☐ 60 + YEARS OF AGE

RESTING ECG   **EXERCISE ECG**
0 ☐ NORMAL 0 ☐
1 ☐ EQUIVOCAL 4 ☐
3 ☐ ABNORMAL 8 ☐

TOTAL CORONARY RISK
☐ VERY LOW (0- 4)
☐ LOW (5-12)
☐ MODERATE (13-21)
☐ HIGH (22-31)
☐ VERY HIGH (32 +)

PREVIOUS TOTAL

COOPER CLINIC/ Dallas, Texas

Coronary Risk Profile

NAME:	**Males: *30-39 Years of Age**

PERCENTILE RANKINGS	BALKE TREADMILL TIME (min.)	TOTAL CHOLESTEROL/ HDL RATIO	TRIGLYCERIDE (mg. %)	GLUCOSE (mg. %)	% BODY FAT	RESTING BLOOD PRESSURE SYSTOLIC (mm HG)	DIASTOLIC (mm HG)
YOUR VALUES							
99	29:00	2.4	35.0	75.0	5.2	94.0	60.0
97	27:00	2.7	43.0	80.0	7.7	100.0	64.0
95	26:00	2.9	47.0	82.0	9.1	100.0	66.0
90	24:30	3.2	56.0	85.0	11.3	104.0	70.0
85	23:00	3.4	63.0	88.0	12.7	108.0	70.0
80	22:00	3.6	69.0	89.0	13.9	110.0	70.0
75	21:00	3.8	75.0	91.0	14.9	110.0	72.0
70	20:30	3.9	80.0	92.0	15.9	112.0	74.0
65	20:00	4.1	87.0	93.0	16.6	114.0	76.0
60	19:00	4.3	92.0	95.0	17.5	116.0	78.0
55	18:25	4.4	98.0	96.0	18.2	118.0	78.0
50	18:00	4.6	105.0	97.0	19.0	120.0	80.0
45	17:00	4.8	112.0	98.0	19.7	120.0	80.0
40	16:32	5.0	121.0	100.0	20.5	120.0	80.0
35	16:00	5.2	130.0	101.0	21.4	122.0	82.0
30	15:30	5.4	142.0	102.0	22.3	124.0	84.0
25	15:00	5.7	157.0	104.0	23.2	128.0	84.0
20	14:06	6.0	176.0	105.0	24.2	130.0	86.0
15	13:10	6.4	200.0	107.0	25.5	132.0	90.0
10	12:09	6.9	235.0	110.0	27.3	136.0	90.0
5	11:00	7.8	304.2	115.0	29.9	140.0	96.0
3	10:00	8.4	365.0	120.0	31.6	145.0	100.0
1	8:00	10.2	548.7	130.0	35.6	154.0	104.0
N	7094	3188	5975	5975	5611	7162	7162

PERSONAL HISTORY OF HEART ATTACK OR BYPASS

- 0 ☐ NONE
- 2 ☐ OVER 5 YEARS AGO
- 4 ☐ 2 - 5 YEARS AGO
- 5 ☐ 1 - < 2 YEARS AGO
- 8 ☐ 0 - < 1 YEAR AGO

FAMILY HISTORY OF CORONARY HEART DISEASE

- 0 ☐ NONE OR OVER 65
- 2 ☐ YES, AGE 50-65
- 4 ☐ YES, UNDER AGE 50

KNOWN CORONARY HEART DISEASE W/O HEART ATTACK OR BYPASS

- 0 ☐ NONE
- 2 ☐ OVER 5 YEARS AGO
- 4 ☐ 2 - 5 YEARS AGO
- 5 ☐ 1 - < 2 YEARS AGO
- 6 ☐ 0 - < 1 YEAR AGO

SMOKING HABITS

- 0 ☐ NONE
- 0 ☐ PAST 1 YEAR OR MORE
- 1 ☐ PAST ONLY LESS THAN 1 YEAR
- 1 ☐ PIPE/CIGAR
- 2 ☐ 1 - 10 DAILY
- 3 ☐ 11 - 20 DAILY
- 4 ☐ 21 - 30 DAILY
- 5 ☐ 31 - 40 DAILY
- 6 ☐ MORE THAN 40 DAILY

TENSION - ANXIETY

- 0 ☐ NO TENSION, VERY RELAXED
- 0 ☐ SLIGHT TENSION
- 1 ☐ MODERATE TENSION
- 2 ☐ HIGH TENSION
- 3 ☐ VERY TENSE, "HIGH STRUNG"

- 3 ☐ DIABETES

*Data based on first visit only
© Institute for Aerobics Research - 1985

AGE FACTOR

- 0 ☐ UNDER 30 YEARS OF AGE
- 1 ☐ 30 - 39 YEARS OF AGE
- 2 ☐ 40 - 49 YEARS OF AGE
- 3 ☐ 50 - 59 YEARS OF AGE
- 4 ☐ 60 + YEARS OF AGE

	RESTING ECG	EXERCISE ECG
0 ☐	NORMAL	0 ☐
1 ☐	EQUIVOCAL	4 ☐
3 ☐	ABNORMAL	8 ☐

TOTAL CORONARY RISK

- ☐ VERY LOW (0- 4)
- ☐ LOW (5-12)
- ☐ MODERATE (13-21)
- ☐ HIGH (22-31)
- ☐ VERY HIGH (32 +)

PREVIOUS TOTAL

COOPER CLINIC/ Dallas, Texas   **Coronary Risk Profile**

NAME:						**Males: *40-49 Years of Age**	

PERCENTILE RANKINGS	BALKE TREADMILL TIME (min.)	TOTAL CHOLESTEROL/ HDL RATIO	TRIGLYCERIDE (mg. %)	GLUCOSE (mg. %)	% BODY FAT	RESTING BLOOD PRESSURE SYSTOLIC (mm HG)	DIASTOLIC (mm HG)
YOUR VALUES							
99	28:00	2.6	38.0	77.0	6.6	94.0	60.0
97	25:45	2.9	47.0	81.0	9.9	100.0	65.0
95	24:30	3.1	53.0	84.0	11.4	100.0	68.0
90	23:00	3.4	63.0	87.0	13.6	106.0	70.0
85	21:00	3.6	70.0	89.0	15.1	110.0	72.0
80	20:10	3.8	77.0	91.0	16.3	110.0	74.0
75	20:00	4.1	84.0	92.0	17.3	112.0	76.0
70	18:32	4.2	90.0	94.0	18.1	114.0	78.0
65	18:00	4.4	97.0	95.0	18.8	116.0	78.0
60	17:15	4.6	104.0	97.0	19.6	118.0	80.0
55	17:00	4.8	111.0	98.0	20.3	120.0	80.0
50	16:00	5.0	119.0	99.0	21.1	120.0	80.0
45	15:30	5.2	128.0	100.0	21.8	120.0	80.0
40	15:00	5.4	138.0	102.0	22.5	122.0	82.0
35	14:15	5.7	149.0	104.0	23.3	124.0	84.0
30	13:57	5.9	162.0	105.0	24.1	128.0	86.0
25	13:00	6.2	177.0	107.0	25.0	130.0	88.0
20	12:30	6.5	199.0	109.0	26.1	130.0	90.0
15	12:00	6.9	226.0	111.0	27.3	135.0	90.0
10	10:59	7.5	263.0	115.0	28.9	140.0	94.0
5	9:13	8.4	360.0	120.0	31.5	146.0	100.0
3	8:00	9.0	420.1	125.0	33.4	150.0	102.0
1	6:21	10.6	656.1	147.1	37.4	160.0	110.0
N	6837	3073	6196	6192	5724	6939	6939

PERSONAL HISTORY OF HEART ATTACK OR BYPASS
0 □ NONE
2 □ OVER 5 YEARS AGO
4 □ 2 - 5 YEARS AGO
5 □ 1 - < 2 YEARS AGO
8 □ 0 - < 1 YEAR AGO

FAMILY HISTORY OF CORONARY HEART DISEASE
0 □ NONE OR OVER 65
2 □ YES, AGE 50-65
4 □ YES, UNDER AGE 50

KNOWN CORONARY HEART DISEASE W/O HEART ATTACK OR BYPASS
0 □ NONE
2 □ OVER 5 YEARS AGO
4 □ 2 - 5 YEARS AGO
5 □ 1 - < 2 YEARS AGO
6 □ 0 - < 1 YEAR AGO

SMOKING HABITS
0 □ NONE
0 □ PAST 1 YEAR OR MORE
1 □ PAST ONLY LESS THAN 1 YEAR
1 □ PIPE/CIGAR
2 □ 1 - 10 DAILY
3 □ 11 - 20 DAILY
4 □ 21 - 30 DAILY
5 □ 31 - 40 DAILY
6 □ MORE THAN 40 DAILY

TENSION - ANXIETY
0 □ NO TENSION, VERY RELAXED
0 □ SLIGHT TENSION
1 □ MODERATE TENSION
2 □ HIGH TENSION
3 □ VERY TENSE, "HIGH STRUNG"

3 □ DIABETES

*Data based on first visit only
® Institute for Aerobics Research - 1985

AGE FACTOR
0 □ UNDER 30 YEARS OF AGE
1 □ 30 - 39 YEARS OF AGE
2 □ 40 - 49 YEARS OF AGE
3 □ 50 - 59 YEARS OF AGE
4 □ 60 + YEARS OF AGE

RESTING ECG		**EXERCISE ECG**
0 □	NORMAL	0 □
1 □	EQUIVOCAL	4 □
3 □	ABNORMAL	8 □

TOTAL CORONARY RISK
□ VERY LOW   (0- 4)
□ LOW   (5-12)
□ MODERATE   (13-21)
□ HIGH   (22-31)
□ VERY HIGH   (32 +)

PREVIOUS TOTAL

| NAME: | | | | | | **Males: *50-59 Years of Age** | |

PERCENTILE RANKINGS	BALKE TREADMILL TIME (min.)	TOTAL CHOLESTEROL/ HDL RATIO	TRIGLYCERIDE (mg. %)	GLUCOSE (mg. %)	% BODY FAT	RESTING BLOOD PRESSURE SYSTOLIC (mm HG)	DIASTOLIC (mm HG)
YOUR VALUES							
99	26:00	2.6	39.0	77.0	8.8	96.0	62.0
97	24:00	2.9	48.0	82.0	11.5	100.0	68.0
95	22:15	3.1	54.0	85.0	12.9	104.0	70.0
90	21:00	3.5	64.0	88.0	15.3	108.0	70.0
85	19:00	3.7	74.0	90.0	16.9	110.0	74.0
80	18:00	4.0	81.0	92.0	17.9	114.0	76.0
75	17:00	4.2	88.0	94.0	19.0	116.0	78.0
70	16:15	4.4	95.0	96.0	19.8	118.0	80.0
65	15:40	4.6	101.0	98.0	20.6	120.0	80.0
60	15:00	4.8	108.0	99.0	21.3	120.0	80.0
55	15:00	5.0	116.0	100.0	22.1	122.0	80.0
50	14:00	5.2	124.0	102.0	22.7	124.0	82.0
45	13:15	5.4	134.0	103.0	23.4	126.0	84.0
40	13:00	5.6	144.0	105.0	24.1	130.0	85.0
35	12:07	5.8	156.0	106.0	24.9	130.0	86.0
30	12:00	6.1	168.0	108.0	25.7	132.0	88.0
25	11:08	6.3	185.0	110.0	26.6	136.0	90.0
20	10:30	6.6	202.0	113.0	27.5	140.0	90.0
15	10:00	7.1	231.0	115.0	28.8	140.0	94.0
10	9:00	7.6	274.0	120.0	30.3	146.0	98.0
5	7:00	8.5	355.6	130.0	32.4	154.0	100.0
3	6:06	9.4	420.0	141.0	33.8	160.0	104.0
1	4:54	11.4	653.2	215.9	38.1	172.0	110.0
N	3808	1811	3567	3577	3275	3984	3984

PERSONAL HISTORY OF HEART ATTACK OR BYPASS
0 ☐ NONE
2 ☐ OVER 5 YEARS AGO
4 ☐ 2 - 5 YEARS AGO
5 ☐ 1 - < 2 YEARS AGO
8 ☐ 0 - < 1 YEAR AGO

FAMILY HISTORY OF CORONARY HEART DISEASE
0 ☐ NONE OR OVER 65
2 ☐ YES, AGE 50-65
4 ☐ YES, UNDER AGE 50

KNOWN CORONARY HEART DISEASE W/O HEART ATTACK OR BYPASS
0 ☐ NONE
2 ☐ OVER 5 YEARS AGO
4 ☐ 2 - 5 YEARS AGO
5 ☐ 1 - < 2 YEARS AGO
6 ☐ 0 - < 1 YEAR AGO

SMOKING HABITS
0 ☐ NONE
0 ☐ PAST 1 YEAR OR MORE
1 ☐ PAST ONLY LESS THAN 1 YEAR
1 ☐ PIPE/CIGAR
2 ☐ 1 - 10 DAILY
3 ☐ 11 - 20 DAILY
4 ☐ 21 - 30 DAILY
5 ☐ 31 - 40 DAILY
6 ☐ MORE THAN 40 DAILY

TENSION - ANXIETY
0 ☐ NO TENSION, VERY RELAXED
0 ☐ SLIGHT TENSION
1 ☐ MODERATE TENSION
2 ☐ HIGH TENSION
3 ☐ VERY TENSE, "HIGH STRUNG"

3 ☐ DIABETES

*Data based on first visit only
© Institute for Aerobics Research - 1985

AGE FACTOR
0 ☐ UNDER 30 YEARS OF AGE
1 ☐ 30 - 39 YEARS OF AGE
2 ☐ 40 - 49 YEARS OF AGE
3 ☐ 50 - 59 YEARS OF AGE
4 ☐ 60 + YEARS OF AGE

RESTING ECG   EXERCISE ECG
0 ☐   NORMAL   0 ☐
1 ☐   EQUIVOCAL   4 ☐
3 ☐   ABNORMAL   8 ☐

TOTAL CORONARY RISK
☐ VERY LOW   (0- 4)
☐ LOW   (5-12)
☐ MODERATE   (13-21)
☐ HIGH   (22-31)
☐ VERY HIGH   (32 +)

PREVIOUS TOTAL

COOPER CLINIC/ Dallas, Texas

Coronary Risk Profile

NAME:

Males: * ≥ 60 Years of Age

PERCENTILE RANKINGS	BALKE TREADMILL TIME (min.)	TOTAL CHOLESTEROL/ HDL RATIO	TRIGLYCERIDE (mg. %)	GLUCOSE (mg. %)	% BODY FAT	RESTING BLOOD PRESSURE SYSTOLIC (mm HG)	DIASTOLIC (mm HG)
YOUR VALUES							
99	24:29	2.5	42.0	74.7	7.7	100.0	60.0
97	22:00	2.9	49.0	82.7	11.7	102.0	66.0
95	20:56	3.1	54.0	85.0	13.1	106.0	68.0
90	19:00	3.3	63.0	89.0	15.3	110.0	70.0
85	17:00	3.6	70.0	91.0	17.2	115.0	72.0
80	16:00	3.7	77.0	93.0	18.4	118.0	74.0
75	15:00	4.0	83.0	95.0	19.3	120.0	78.0
70	14:04	4.2	89.0	96.0	20.3	120.0	78.0
65	13:22	4.4	97.0	98.0	21.1	124.0	80.0
60	12:53	4.6	105.0	100.0	22.0	126.0	80.0
55	12:03	4.7	112.5	101.0	22.6	130.0	80.0
50	11:40	5.0	120.0	103.0	23.5	130.0	82.0
45	11:00	5.2	129.0	105.0	24.3	132.0	84.0
40	10:30	5.4	140.0	107.0	25.0	136.0	85.0
35	10:00	5.7	150.0	108.5	25.9	140.0	88.0
30	9:30	5.9	163.0	110.0	26.7	140.0	90.0
25	8:54	6.2	177.0	113.0	27.6	144.0	90.0
20	8:00	6.4	194.0	115.0	28.5	148.0	90.2
15	7:00	6.7	216.0	119.0	29.7	150.0	94.0
10	5:35	7.1	250.0	124.0	31.2	160.0	98.0
5	4:00	8.0	307.5	137.5	33.4	168.0	100.0
3	3:30	8.4	362.6	149.3	35.1	172.5	105.5
1	2:17	9.6	464.9	179.0	41.3	185.6	112.0
N	1005	570	1089	1089	984	1258	1258

PERSONAL HISTORY OF HEART ATTACK OR BYPASS

- 0 ☐ NONE
- 2 ☐ OVER 5 YEARS AGO
- 4 ☐ 2 - 5 YEARS AGO
- 5 ☐ 1 - < 2 YEARS AGO
- 8 ☐ 0 - < 1 YEAR AGO

FAMILY HISTORY OF CORONARY HEART DISEASE

- 0 ☐ NONE OR OVER 65
- 2 ☐ YES, AGE 50-65
- 4 ☐ YES, UNDER AGE 50

KNOWN CORONARY HEART DISEASE W/O HEART ATTACK OR BYPASS

- 0 ☐ NONE
- 2 ☐ OVER 5 YEARS AGO
- 4 ☐ 2 - 5 YEARS AGO
- 5 ☐ 1 - < 2 YEARS AGO
- 6 ☐ 0 - < 1 YEAR AGO

SMOKING HABITS

- 0 ☐ NONE
- 0 ☐ PAST 1 YEAR OR MORE
- 1 ☐ PAST ONLY LESS THAN 1 YEAR
- 1 ☐ PIPE/CIGAR
- 2 ☐ 1 - 10 DAILY
- 3 ☐ 11 - 20 DAILY
- 4 ☐ 21 - 30 DAILY
- 5 ☐ 31 - 40 DAILY
- 6 ☐ MORE THAN 40 DAILY

TENSION - ANXIETY

- 0 ☐ NO TENSION, VERY RELAXED
- 0 ☐ SLIGHT TENSION
- 1 ☐ MODERATE TENSION
- 2 ☐ HIGH TENSION
- 3 ☐ VERY TENSE, "HIGH STRUNG"

- 3 ☐ DIABETES

*Data based on first visit only
© Institute for Aerobics Research - 1985

AGE FACTOR

- 0 ☐ UNDER 30 YEARS OF AGE
- 1 ☐ 30 - 39 YEARS OF AGE
- 2 ☐ 40 - 49 YEARS OF AGE
- 3 ☐ 50 - 59 YEARS OF AGE
- 4 ☐ 60 + YEARS OF AGE

RESTING ECG   EXERCISE ECG

- 0 ☐   NORMAL   0 ☐
- 1 ☐   EQUIVOCAL   4 ☐
- 3 ☐   ABNORMAL   8 ☐

TOTAL CORONARY RISK

- ☐ VERY LOW   (0- 4)
- ☐ LOW   (5-12)
- ☐ MODERATE   (13-21)
- ☐ HIGH   (22-31)
- ☐ VERY HIGH   (32 +)

PREVIOUS TOTAL

COOPER CLINIC/ Dallas, Texas

Coronary Risk Profile

NAME:						Females: * < 30 Years of Age	

PERCENTILE RANKINGS	BALKE TREADMILL TIME (min.)	TOTAL CHOLESTEROL/ HDL RATIO	TRIGLYCERIDE (mg. %)	GLUCOSE (mg. %)	% BODY FAT	RESTING BLOOD PRESSURE SYSTOLIC (mm HG)	DIASTOLIC (mm HG)
YOUR VALUES							
99	26:21	2.0	30.0	64.7	5.4	84.0	53.7
97	23:24	2.2	33.0	72.7	9.3	90.0	58.0
95	22:00	2.3	36.0	75.0	10.8	90.0	60.0
90	20:12	2.4	42.0	78.0	14.5	92.0	60.0
85	19:00	2.6	45.0	80.0	16.0	96.0	62.0
80	18:00	2.7	48.0	81.0	17.1	99.2	64.0
75	17:00	2.8	50.0	83.0	18.2	100.0	66.0
70	16:00	2.9	54.0	85.0	19.0	100.0	68.0
65	15:30	2.9	57.0	85.0	19.8	102.0	68.0
60	15:00	3.1	60.0	87.0	20.6	104.0	70.0
55	14:39	3.1	64.0	88.0	21.3	106.0	70.0
50	14:00	3.2	67.0	89.0	22.1	108.0	70.0
45	13:30	3.3	72.0	90.0	22.7	110.0	70.0
40	13:00	3.4	75.0	91.0	23.7	110.0	72.0
35	12:17	3.5	79.0	92.0	24.4	111.9	74.0
30	12:00	3.6	85.0	94.0	25.4	112.0	76.0
25	11:03	3.8	92.0	95.0	26.6	115.0	78.0
20	10:50	3.9	101.0	97.0	27.7	118.0	78.8
15	10:00	4.1	110.6	99.0	29.8	120.0	80.0
10	9:17	4.4	133.0	100.0	32.1	120.0	80.0
5	7:33	4.9	162.9	105.0	35.4	128.0	86.0
3	6:45	5.4	202.2	107.0	37.2	130.0	89.0
1	5:15	6.2	279.9	119.8	40.5	140.0	90.0
N	764	372	622	623	638	782	782

PERSONAL HISTORY OF HEART ATTACK OR BYPASS
0 ☐ NONE
2 ☐ OVER 5 YEARS AGO
4 ☐ 2 - 5 YEARS AGO
5 ☐ 1 - < 2 YEARS AGO
8 ☐ 0 - < 1 YEAR AGO

FAMILY HISTORY OF CORONARY HEART DISEASE
0 ☐ NONE OR OVER 65
2 ☐ YES, AGE 50-65
4 ☐ YES, UNDER AGE 50

KNOWN CORONARY HEART DISEASE W/O HEART ATTACK OR BYPASS
0 ☐ NONE
2 ☐ OVER 5 YEARS AGO
4 ☐ 2 - 5 YEARS AGO
5 ☐ 1 - < 2 YEARS AGO
6 ☐ 0 - < 1 YEAR AGO

SMOKING HABITS
0 ☐ NONE
0 ☐ PAST 1 YEAR OR MORE
1 ☐ PAST ONLY LESS THAN 1 YEAR
1 ☐ PIPE/CIGAR
2 ☐ 1 - 10 DAILY
3 ☐ 11 - 20 DAILY
4 ☐ 21 - 30 DAILY
5 ☐ 31 - 40 DAILY
6 ☐ MORE THAN 40 DAILY

TENSION - ANXIETY
0 ☐ NO TENSION, VERY RELAXED
0 ☐ SLIGHT TENSION
1 ☐ MODERATE TENSION
2 ☐ HIGH TENSION
3 ☐ VERY TENSE, "HIGH STRUNG"

3 ☐ DIABETES

*Data based on first visit only
© Institute for Aerobics Research - 1985

AGE FACTOR
0 ☐ UNDER 30 YEARS OF AGE
1 ☐ 30 - 39 YEARS OF AGE
2 ☐ 40 - 49 YEARS OF AGE
3 ☐ 50 - 59 YEARS OF AGE
4 ☐ 60 + YEARS OF AGE

RESTING ECG		EXERCISE ECG
0 ☐	NORMAL	0 ☐
1 ☐	EQUIVOCAL	4 ☐
3 ☐	ABNORMAL	8 ☐

TOTAL CORONARY RISK
☐ VERY LOW (0- 4)
☐ LOW (5-12)
☐ MODERATE (13-21)
☐ HIGH (22-31)
☐ VERY HIGH (32 +)

PREVIOUS TOTAL

NAME: **Females: *30-39 Years of Age**

PERCENTILE RANKINGS	BALKE TREADMILL TIME (min.)	TOTAL CHOLESTEROL/ HDL RATIO	TRIGLYCERIDE (mg. %)	GLUCOSE (mg. %)	% BODY FAT	RESTING BLOOD PRESSURE SYSTOLIC (mm HG)	DIASTOLIC (mm HG)
YOUR VALUES							
99	23:22	1.9	24.9	69.0	7.3	86.0	54.0
97	21:00	2.1	31.0	75.0	11.0	90.0	60.0
95	20:00	2.2	35.0	77.0	13.4	90.0	60.0
90	18:00	2.4	40.0	81.0	15.5	94.0	62.0
85	17:30	2.6	43.0	83.0	16.9	98.0	64.0
80	16:20	2.7	47.0	84.0	18.0	100.0	66.0
75	15:30	2.7	50.0	85.0	19.1	100.0	68.0
70	15:00	2.8	52.0	87.0	20.0	100.1	70.0
65	14:10	2.9	55.0	88.0	20.8	102.0	70.0
60	13:35	3.0	59.0	89.0	21.6	104.0	70.0
55	13:00	3.1	62.0	90.0	22.4	106.0	70.0
50	13:00	3.1	66.0	91.0	23.1	108.0	72.0
45	12:00	3.2	69.0	92.0	24.0	110.0	74.0
40	12:00	3.3	73.0	94.0	24.9	110.0	75.0
35	11:09	3.4	78.0	95.0	26.0	112.0	76.0
30	10:45	3.5	82.0	96.0	27.0	114.0	78.0
25	10:00	3.7	87.0	97.0	28.1	116.0	80.0
20	9:30	3.9	93.0	99.0	29.3	120.0	80.0
15	9:00	4.1	102.0	101.0	31.0	120.0	80.0
10	8:00	4.4	117.0	104.0	32.8	124.0	84.0
5	7:00	4.7	144.0	107.3	35.7	130.0	90.0
3	6:10	5.1	163.0	110.2	37.5	138.0	90.0
1	5:12	6.2	222.0	119.0	40.0	145.0	98.0
N	2049	799	1392	1394	1336	2096	2096

PERSONAL HISTORY OF HEART ATTACK OR BYPASS
- 0 ☐ NONE
- 2 ☐ OVER 5 YEARS AGO
- 4 ☐ 2 - 5 YEARS AGO
- 5 ☐ 1 - < 2 YEARS AGO
- 8 ☐ 0 - < 1 YEAR AGO

FAMILY HISTORY OF CORONARY HEART DISEASE
- 0 ☐ NONE OR OVER 65
- 2 ☐ YES, AGE 50-65
- 4 ☐ YES, UNDER AGE 50

KNOWN CORONARY HEART DISEASE W/O HEART ATTACK OR BYPASS
- 0 ☐ NONE
- 2 ☐ OVER 5 YEARS AGO
- 4 ☐ 2 - 5 YEARS AGO
- 5 ☐ 1 - < 2 YEARS AGO
- 6 ☐ 0 - < 1 YEAR AGO

SMOKING HABITS
- 0 ☐ NONE
- 0 ☐ PAST 1 YEAR OR MORE
- 1 ☐ PAST ONLY LESS THAN 1 YEAR
- 1 ☐ PIPE/CIGAR
- 2 ☐ 1 - 10 DAILY
- 3 ☐ 11 - 20 DAILY
- 4 ☐ 21 - 30 DAILY
- 5 ☐ 31 - 40 DAILY
- 6 ☐ MORE THAN 40 DAILY

TENSION - ANXIETY
- 0 ☐ NO TENSION, VERY RELAXED
- 0 ☐ SLIGHT TENSION
- 1 ☐ MODERATE TENSION
- 2 ☐ HIGH TENSION
- 3 ☐ VERY TENSE, "HIGH STRUNG"
- 3 ☐ DIABETES

*Data based on first visit only
℮ Institute for Aerobics Research - 1985

AGE FACTOR
- 0 ☐ UNDER 30 YEARS OF AGE
- 1 ☐ 30 - 39 YEARS OF AGE
- 2 ☐ 40 - 49 YEARS OF AGE
- 3 ☐ 50 - 59 YEARS OF AGE
- 4 ☐ 60 + YEARS OF AGE

RESTING ECG   **EXERCISE ECG**
		RESTING	EXERCISE
	NORMAL	0 ☐	0 ☐
	EQUIVOCAL	1 ☐	4 ☐
	ABNORMAL	3 ☐	8 ☐

TOTAL CORONARY RISK
- ☐ VERY LOW   (0- 4)
- ☐ LOW   (5-12)
- ☐ MODERATE   (13-21)
- ☐ HIGH   (22-31)
- ☐ VERY HIGH   (32 +)

PREVIOUS TOTAL

COOPER CLINIC/ Dallas, Texas

Coronary Risk Profile

NAME:

Females: *40-49 Years of Age

PERCENTILE RANKINGS	BALKE TREADMILL TIME (min.)	TOTAL CHOLESTEROL/ HDL RATIO	TRIGLYCERIDE (mg. %)	GLUCOSE (mg. %)	% BODY FAT	RESTING BLOOD PRESSURE SYSTOLIC (mm HG)	DIASTOLIC (mm HG)
YOUR VALUES							
99	22:00	2.0	29.0	73.0	11.6	85.2	58.0
97	20:00	2.2	35.0	76.4	14.1	90.0	60.0
95	18:00	2.4	39.0	78.0	16.1	92.0	60.2
90	17:00	2.6	44.0	82.0	18.5	96.0	65.0
85	15:35	2.7	48.0	84.0	20.3	100.0	68.0
80	14:45	2.8	52.0	85.4	21.3	100.0	70.0
75	13:56	2.9	56.0	87.0	22.4	102.0	70.0
70	13:00	2.9	60.0	89.0	23.5	104.0	70.0
65	12:30	3.1	63.0	90.0	24.3	106.0	72.0
60	12:00	3.1	67.0	91.0	24.9	110.0	74.0
55	11:30	3.2	71.0	92.0	25.5	110.0	75.0
50	11:00	3.4	74.0	93.0	26.4	110.0	76.0
45	10:48	3.5	79.0	94.0	27.3	112.0	78.0
40	10:01	3.6	85.0	95.0	28.1	114.0	80.0
35	10:00	3.7	91.0	96.0	29.0	118.0	80.0
30	9:11	3.9	98.0	98.0	30.1	120.0	80.0
25	9:00	4.0	106.0	100.0	31.1	120.0	80.0
20	8:00	4.2	116.0	101.0	32.1	122.0	82.0
15	7:20	4.5	130.0	104.0	33.3	128.0	84.0
10	7:00	4.8	149.0	107.0	35.0	130.0	88.0
5	5:55	5.4	185.0	111.0	37.8	139.8	92.0
3	5:00	5.8	221.1	115.0	39.1	140.3	96.0
1	4:00	7.3	317.0	125.5	45.5	152.0	104.0
N	1630	757	1348	1346	1175	1761	1761

PERSONAL HISTORY OF HEART ATTACK OR BYPASS
0 ☐ NONE
2 ☐ OVER 5 YEARS AGO
4 ☐ 2 - 5 YEARS AGO
5 ☐ 1 - < 2 YEARS AGO
8 ☐ 0 - < 1 YEAR AGO

FAMILY HISTORY OF CORONARY HEART DISEASE
0 ☐ NONE OR OVER 65
2 ☐ YES, AGE 50-65
4 ☐ YES, UNDER AGE 50

KNOWN CORONARY HEART DISEASE W/O HEART ATTACK OR BYPASS
0 ☐ NONE
2 ☐ OVER 5 YEARS AGO
4 ☐ 2 - 5 YEARS AGO
5 ☐ 1 - < 2 YEARS AGO
6 ☐ 0 - < 1 YEAR AGO

SMOKING HABITS
0 ☐ NONE
0 ☐ PAST 1 YEAR OR MORE
1 ☐ PAST ONLY LESS THAN 1 YEAR
1 ☐ PIPE/CIGAR
2 ☐ 1 - 10 DAILY
3 ☐ 11 - 20 DAILY
4 ☐ 21 - 30 DAILY
5 ☐ 31 - 40 DAILY
6 ☐ MORE THAN 40 DAILY

TENSION - ANXIETY
0 ☐ NO TENSION, VERY RELAXED
0 ☐ SLIGHT TENSION
1 ☐ MODERATE TENSION
2 ☐ HIGH TENSION
3 ☐ VERY TENSE, "HIGH STRUNG"

3 ☐ DIABETES

*Data based on first visit only
© Institute for Aerobics Research - 1985

AGE FACTOR
0 ☐ UNDER 30 YEARS OF AGE
1 ☐ 30 - 39 YEARS OF AGE
2 ☐ 40 - 49 YEARS OF AGE
3 ☐ 50 - 59 YEARS OF AGE
4 ☐ 60 + YEARS OF AGE

RESTING ECG   EXERCISE ECG
0 ☐ NORMAL 0 ☐
1 ☐ EQUIVOCAL 4 ☐
3 ☐ ABNORMAL 8 ☐

TOTAL CORONARY RISK
☐ VERY LOW (0- 4)
☐ LOW (5-12)
☐ MODERATE (13-21)
☐ HIGH (22-31)
☐ VERY HIGH (32 +)

PREVIOUS TOTAL

COOPER CLINIC / Dallas, Texas

Coronary Risk Profile

NAME:

Females: *50-59 Years of Age

PERCENTILE RANKINGS	BALKE TREADMILL TIME (min.)	TOTAL CHOLESTEROL/ HDL RATIO	TRIGLYCERIDE (mg. %)	GLUCOSE (mg. %)	% BODY FAT	RESTING BLOOD PRESSURE SYSTOLIC (mm HG)	RESTING BLOOD PRESSURE DIASTOLIC (mm HG)
YOUR VALUES							
99	18:44	2.2	35.0	73.0	11.6	90.0	60.0
97	16:00	2.5	41.0	78.7	16.6	94.0	62.0
95	15:07	2.6	47.0	81.0	18.8	98.0	64.0
90	14:00	2.7	54.0	84.0	21.6	100.0	70.0
85	12:53	2.8	60.0	86.4	23.6	104.0	70.0
80	12:00	3.0	66.0	88.0	25.0	108.0	70.0
75	11:43	3.2	70.0	90.0	25.8	110.0	72.0
70	11:00	3.3	75.0	92.0	26.6	110.0	74.0
65	10:14	3.4	81.0	93.0	27.4	114.0	76.0
60	10:00	3.5	87.0	94.0	28.5	116.0	78.0
55	9:30	3.6	92.0	96.0	29.2	120.0	80.0
50	9:10	3.7	99.0	97.0	30.1	120.0	80.0
45	9:00	3.8	106.0	98.0	30.8	120.7	80.0
40	8:13	4.0	112.8	100.0	31.6	124.0	80.0
35	7:43	4.1	121.0	101.0	32.6	126.0	82.0
30	7:16	4.3	127.0	103.0	33.5	130.0	84.0
25	7:00	4.5	138.0	105.0	34.3	132.0	86.0
20	6:25	4.8	155.0	106.0	35.6	136.0	88.0
15	6:00	5.0	166.0	110.0	36.6	140.0	90.0
10	5:05	5.4	187.7	113.0	37.9	146.0	94.0
5	4:14	6.2	223.4	121.0	39.6	160.0	100.0
3	3:58	6.6	245.2	130.0	40.8	164.0	101.0
1	2:36	7.6	357.0	181.4	50.8	180.0	112.3
N	878	467	892	888	708	1082	1082

PERSONAL HISTORY OF HEART ATTACK OR BYPASS

0 ☐ NONE
2 ☐ OVER 5 YEARS AGO
4 ☐ 2 - 5 YEARS AGO
5 ☐ 1 - < 2 YEARS AGO
8 ☐ 0 - < 1 YEAR AGO

FAMILY HISTORY OF CORONARY HEART DISEASE

0 ☐ NONE OR OVER 65
2 ☐ YES, AGE 50-65
4 ☐ YES, UNDER AGE 50

KNOWN CORONARY HEART DISEASE W/O HEART ATTACK OR BYPASS

0 ☐ NONE
2 ☐ OVER 5 YEARS AGO
4 ☐ 2 - 5 YEARS AGO
5 ☐ 1 - < 2 YEARS AGO
6 ☐ 0 - < 1 YEAR AGO

SMOKING HABITS

0 ☐ NONE
0 ☐ PAST 1 YEAR OR MORE
1 ☐ PAST ONLY LESS THAN 1 YEAR
1 ☐ PIPE/CIGAR
2 ☐ 1 - 10 DAILY
3 ☐ 11 - 20 DAILY
4 ☐ 21 - 30 DAILY
5 ☐ 31 - 40 DAILY
6 ☐ MORE THAN 40 DAILY

TENSION - ANXIETY

0 ☐ NO TENSION, VERY RELAXED
0 ☐ SLIGHT TENSION
1 ☐ MODERATE TENSION
2 ☐ HIGH TENSION
3 ☐ VERY TENSE, "HIGH STRUNG"

3 ☐ DIABETES

*Data based on first visit only
© Institute for Aerobics Research - 1985

AGE FACTOR

0 ☐ UNDER 30 YEARS OF AGE
1 ☐ 30 - 39 YEARS OF AGE
2 ☐ 40 - 49 YEARS OF AGE
3 ☐ 50 - 59 YEARS OF AGE
4 ☐ 60 + YEARS OF AGE

RESTING ECG		EXERCISE ECG
0 ☐	NORMAL	0 ☐
1 ☐	EQUIVOCAL	4 ☐
3 ☐	ABNORMAL	8 ☐

TOTAL CORONARY RISK

☐ VERY LOW (0- 4)
☐ LOW (5-12)
☐ MODERATE (13-21)
☐ HIGH (22-31)
☐ VERY HIGH (32 +)

PREVIOUS TOTAL

COOPER CLINIC/ Dallas, Texas

Coronary Risk Profile

NAME:							
						Females: * ≥60 Years of Age	

PERCENTILE RANKINGS	BALKE TREADMILL TIME (min.)	TOTAL CHOLESTEROL/ HDL RATIO	TRIGLYCERIDE (mg. %)	GLUCOSE (mg. %)	% BODY FAT	RESTING BLOOD PRESSURE SYSTOLIC (mm HG)	DIASTOLIC (mm HG)
YOUR VALUES							
99	20:25	2.0	34.0	77.0	5.4	90.0	58.0
97	16:20	2.6	42.6	80.5	14.8	94.0	60.0
95	15:34	2.6	47.0	84.0	16.8	98.0	64.0
90	14:00	2.8	56.2	86.0	21.1	106.0	70.0
85	12:00	3.0	63.0	88.0	23.5	110.0	70.0
80	11:15	3.1	71.0	89.0	25.1	114.0	72.0
75	11:00	3.2	78.0	91.0	26.7	118.0	74.0
70	10:00	3.4	84.0	92.0	27.5	120.0	76.0
65	9:00	3.5	89.2	93.0	28.5	120.0	78.0
60	8:28	3.6	93.8	94.0	29.3	124.0	78.0
55	8:00	3.9	102.4	95.0	29.9	126.0	80.0
50	7:30	4.1	110.0	97.0	30.9	128.0	80.0
45	7:00	4.2	114.0	99.0	31.8	130.0	80.0
40	6:35	4.4	122.0	100.0	32.5	132.0	82.0
35	6:16	4.6	130.8	102.2	33.0	136.0	84.0
30	6:00	4.8	139.0	104.0	34.3	138.0	86.0
25	6:00	5.0	146.0	106.0	35.5	140.0	88.0
20	5:24	5.2	165.6	108.8	36.6	144.0	90.0
15	5:00	5.4	181.4	110.0	38.0	150.0	90.0
10	4:00	6.0	204.6	114.0	39.3	154.0	94.0
5	3:15	6.6	226.8	123.8	40.5	160.0	100.0
3	2:46	7.5	279.7	139.5	41.4	175.9	100.0
1	2:00	9.2	419.4	180.2	47.0	182.0	105.0
N	202	194	351	350	250	401	401

PERSONAL HISTORY OF HEART ATTACK OR BYPASS
0 ☐ NONE
2 ☐ OVER 5 YEARS AGO
4 ☐ 2 - 5 YEARS AGO
5 ☐ 1 - < 2 YEARS AGO
8 ☐ 0 - < 1 YEAR AGO

FAMILY HISTORY OF CORONARY HEART DISEASE
0 ☐ NONE OR OVER 65
2 ☐ YES, AGE 50-65
4 ☐ YES, UNDER AGE 50

KNOWN CORONARY HEART DISEASE W/O HEART ATTACK OR BYPASS
0 ☐ NONE
2 ☐ OVER 5 YEARS AGO
4 ☐ 2 - 5 YEARS AGO
5 ☐ 1 - < 2 YEARS AGO
6 ☐ 0 - < 1 YEAR AGO

SMOKING HABITS
0 ☐ NONE
0 ☐ PAST 1 YEAR OR MORE
1 ☐ PAST ONLY LESS THAN 1 YEAR
1 ☐ PIPE/CIGAR
2 ☐ 1 - 10 DAILY
3 ☐ 11 - 20 DAILY
4 ☐ 21 - 30 DAILY
5 ☐ 31 - 40 DAILY
6 ☐ MORE THAN 40 DAILY

TENSION - ANXIETY
0 ☐ NO TENSION, VERY RELAXED
0 ☐ SLIGHT TENSION
1 ☐ MODERATE TENSION
2 ☐ HIGH TENSION
3 ☐ VERY TENSE, "HIGH STRUNG"

3 ☐ DIABETES

*Data based on first visit only
© Institute for Aerobics Research - 1985

AGE FACTOR
0 ☐ UNDER 30 YEARS OF AGE
1 ☐ 30 - 39 YEARS OF AGE
2 ☐ 40 - 49 YEARS OF AGE
3 ☐ 50 - 59 YEARS OF AGE
4 ☐ 60 + YEARS OF AGE

	RESTING ECG		EXERCISE ECG
0 ☐	NORMAL		0 ☐
1 ☐	EQUIVOCAL		4 ☐
3 ☐	ABNORMAL		8 ☐

TOTAL CORONARY RISK
☐ VERY LOW (0- 4)
☐ LOW (5-12)
☐ MODERATE (13-21)
☐ HIGH (22-31)
☐ VERY HIGH (32 +)

PREVIOUS TOTAL

SELECTED
REFERENCES

Chapter One

American Medical Association. Special Advertising Supplement, *Newsweek*, 1984.

Fixx, James F. *The Complete Book of Running.* New York: Random House, 1977.

———. *Jackpot!* New York: Random House, 1982.

———. *Jim Fixx's Second Book of Running.* New York: Random House, 1978, 1979, 1980.

Gallup, G. "Runners Extend Distances As Jogging Levels Off." Los Angeles Times Syndicate, January 1983.

———. "Six in Ten Exercise Daily—Remarkable Trend in American Lifestyle." Los Angeles Times Syndicate, June 1984.

Thomas, Gregory S., et al. *Exercise and Health.* Cambridge, Mass.: Oelgeschlager, Gunn & Hain, 1981.

Chapter Two

Cooper, Kenneth H., M.D. "Jim Fixx—Author, Runner, Legend." *Aerobics*, Vol. 5, No. 8, August 1984.

DeYoung, H. Garrett. "State of the Heart." *High Technology,* May 1984.

Henry, Walter L., M.D., et al. "Differences in Distribution of Myocardial Abnormalities in Patients with Obstructive and Nonobstructive Asymmetric Septal Hypertrophy (ASH)." *Circulation,* Vol. 50, September 1974.

Hood, Robert. "Running On." *Scouting,* September 1984.

"James F. Fixx Dies Jogging; Author on Running Was Fifty-two." *The New York Times,* July 22, 1984.

"James Fixx: The Enigma of Heart Disease." *The New York Times,* July 24, 1984.

"Keeping Fit for Life." *Newsweek,* August 6, 1984.

Michener, James A. "Living with an Ailing Heart." *The New York Times Magazine,* August 19, 1984.

Noakes, T. D., et al. "Hypertrophic Cardiomyopathy Associated with Sudden Death During Marathon Racing." *British Heart Journal,* 1979.

Noakes, T. D., M.D., and Rose, A. G., M.D. "Exercise-related Deaths in Subjects with Coexistent Hypertrophic Cardiomyopathy and Coronary Artery Disease." *SA Medical Journal,* Vol. 66, August 1984.

Palmer, Lillis. "Letters to the Editor." *The New York Times Magazine,* September 16, 1984.

Pietschmann, Richard. "Probing Death on the Run." *Runner's World,* November 1984.

Rose, A. G. "Evaluation of Pathological Criteria for Diagnosis of Hypertrophic Cardiomyopathy." *Histopathology,* 1984.

"Why Joggers are Running Scared." *Time,* August 6, 1984.

Woodley, Richard. "Jim Fixx: A Remembrance, a Final Interview." *Official Spectator's Guide, New York City Marathon.* Advertising Supplement to *The New York Times,* 1984.

Zarling, Edwin J., M.D., et al. "Failure to Diagnose Acute Myocardial Infarction." *Journal of the American Medical Association,* Vol. 250, No. 9, September 2, 1983.

Chapter Three

Alpert, Joseph S., M.D. "Association Between Arrhythmias and Mitral Valve Prolapse." *Archives of Internal Medicine,* Vol. 144, December 1984.

Appenzeller, Otto, M.D., and Atkinson, Ruth, M.D. *Sports Medicine.* Baltimore: Urban & Schwarzenberg, 1983.

Cantwell, John D., M.D. "Hypertrophic Cardiomyopathy and the Athlete." *The Physician and Sportsmedicine*, Vol. 12, No. 9, September 1984.

Constant, Richard R., M.D. "Barlow's (The Click) Syndrome." *Aerobics*, Vol. 4, No. 10, October 1983.

Gibbons, Larry W., M.D., et al. "The Acute Cardiac Risk of Strenuous Exercise." *Journal of the American Medical Association*, Vol. 244, No. 16, October 17, 1980.

Jones, Richard J., M.D. "Mortality of Joggers." *Journal of the American Medical Association*, Vol. 247, No. 18, May 14, 1982.

Kannel, William B., M.D., and Abbott, Robert D., Ph.D. "Incidence and Prognosis of Unrecognized Myocardial Infarction." *New England Journal of Medicine*, Vol. 311, No. 18, November 1, 1984.

Kramer, Harvey M., M.D., et al. "Arrhythmias in Mitral Valve Prolapse." *Archives of Internal Medicine*, Vol. 144, December 1984.

Maranto, Gina. "Exercise: How Much Is Too Much?" *Discover*, October 1984.

Ragosta, Michael. "Death During Recreational Exercise in the State of Rhode Island." *Medicine and Science in Sports and Exercise*, Vol. 16, No. 4, 1984.

Siscovick, David S., M.D., et al. "Physical Activity and Primary Cardiac Arrest." *Journal of the American Medical Association*, Vol. 248, No. 23, December 17, 1982.

Thompson, Paul D., M.D. "Incidence of Death During Jogging in Rhode Island from 1975 Through 1980." *Journal of the American Medical Association*, Vol. 247, No. 18, May 14, 1982.

Chapter Four

Bassler, Thomas J., M.D. "Hazards of Restrictive Diets." Letters, *Journal of the American Medical Association*, Vol. 252, No. 4, July 27, 1984.

Benowitz, Neal L., M.D., et al. "Smokers of Low-Yield Cigarettes Do Not Consume Less Nicotine." *New England Journal of Medicine*, Vol. 309, No. 3, July 21, 1983.

Blair, Steven N., et al. "Changes in Coronary Heart Disease Risk Factors Associated with Increased Treadmill Time in 753 Men." *American Journal of Epidemiology*, Vol. 118, No. 3, 1983.

Blair, Steven N., PED, et al. "Physical Fitness and Incidence of Hypertension in Healthy Normotensive Men and Women." *Journal of the American Medical Association*, Vol. 252, No. 4, July 27, 1984.

Bunch, Thomas W., M.D. "Blood Test Abnormalities in Runners." *Mayo Clinic Proceedings,* Vol. 55, February 1980.

Campeau, Lucien, M.D., et al. "The Relation of Risk Factors to the Development of Atherosclerosis in Saphenous Vein Bypass Grafts and the Progression of Disease in the Native Circulation." *New England Journal of Medicine,* Vol. 311, No. 21, November 22, 1984.

"Cholesterol-Heart Disease Link Illuminated." *Science,* Vol. 221, September 1983.

Clegg, Reed S., M.D. "Tarahumara Indians." *Rocky Mountain Medical Journal,* Vol. 69, January 1972.

Connor, William E., M.D., et al. "The Plasma Lipids, Lipoproteins, and Diet of the Tarahumara Indians of Mexico." *American Journal of Clinical Nutrition,* Vol. 31, July 1978.

Cooper, Kenneth H., M.D. " 'Type C' Behavior Patterns." *Aerobics,* Vol. 5, No. 9, September 1984.

"Coronary Risk Factor Intervention Trial—Conclusions and Concerns." *Internal Medicine Alert,* Vol. 4, No. 19, October 11, 1982.

Deanfield, John, et al. "Cigarette Smoking and the Treatment of Angina with Propranolol, Atenolol, and Nifedipine." *New England Journal of Medicine,* Vol. 310, No. 15, April 12, 1984.

"Diet, Drug Treatments Offer Answers to High Cholesterol." *Nutrition & Health News,* Vol. 1, No. 1, Fall 1983.

Duffield, R. G. M., et al. "Treatment of Hyperlipidaemia Retards Progression of Symptomatic Femoral Atherosclerosis." *Lancet,* September 17, 1983.

Ebert, Richard V., M.D., and McNabb, McKendree E., M.D. "Cessation of Smoking in Prevention and Treatment of Cardiac and Pulmonary Disease." Editorials, *Archives of Internal Medicine,* Vol. 144, August 1984.

"Exercise Aids Women on the Pill." *Dallas Times-Herald,* February 26, 1981.

"Exercise to Control Hypertension." *Internal Medicine Alert,* Vol. 6, No. 22, November 30, 1984.

"Fitness Assessment and Development." *Nutrition & Health News,* Vol. II, No. 1, Fall 1984.

Friedman, Meyer, M.D., et al. "Feasibility of Altering Type A Behavior Pattern After Myocardial Infarction." *Circulation,* Vol. 66, No. 1, July 1982.

Goldberg, Linn, M.D., et al. "Changes in Lipid and Lipoprotein Levels After Weight Training." *Journal of the American Medical Association,* Vol. 252, No. 4, July 27, 1984.

Groom, Dale, M.D. "Cardiovascular Observations on Tarahumara Indian Runners—The Modern Spartans." *American Heart Journal,* Vol. 81, No. 3, March 1971.

Hagan, R. Donald, et al. "High Density Lipoprotein Cholesterol in Relation to Food Consumption and Running Distance." *Preventive Medicine,* Vol. 12, 1983.

Hartung, G. Harley, Ph.D., et al. "Effect of Alcohol Intake on High-Density Lipoprotein Cholesterol Levels in Runners and Inactive Men." *Journal of the American Medical Association,* Vol. 249, No. 6, February 11, 1983.

Hartung, G. Harley, Ph.D., et al. "Relation of Diet to High-Density Lipoprotein Cholesterol in Middle-Aged Marathon Runners, Joggers and Inactive Men." *New England Journal of Medicine,* February 14, 1980.

Hartz, Arthur J., M.D., et al. "The Association of Smoking With Cardiomyopathy." *New England Journal of Medicine,* Vol. 311, No. 19, November 8, 1984.

Haskell, William L., Ph.D., et al. "The Effect of Cessation and Resumption of Moderate Alcohol Intake on Serum High-Density Lipoprotein Subfractions." *New England Journal of Medicine,* Vol. 310, No. 13, March 29, 1984.

Haskell, William L., Ph.D. "The Influence of Exercise on the Concentrations of Triglyceride and Cholesterol in Human Plasma."

"Hazards of Cholesterol Proved in Study." *Dallas Times-Herald,* January 18, 1984.

"High Plasma Insulin Level a Prime Risk Factor for Heart Disease." *Journal of the American Medical Association,* Vol. 241, No. 16, April 20, 1979.

Hjalmarson, Agneta I., Ph.D. "Effect of Nicotine Chewing Gum in Smoking Cessation." *Journal of the American Medical Association,* Vol. 252, No. 20, November 23/30, 1984.

"Hold the Eggs and Butter." *Time,* March 26, 1984.

Holmes, T. H., and Rahe, R. H. "The Social Readjustment Rating Scale." *Journal of Psychosomatic Research,* Vol. 11, 1967. Complete wording of Table 3, page 216.

"How Good is 'Good' Cholesterol?" *The Health Letter,* Vol. 19, No. 7, April 9, 1982.

Hubert, Helen B., M.P.H., Ph.D., et al. "Obesity As an Independent Risk Factor for Cardiovascular Disease: A 26-Year Follow-up of Participants in the Framingham Heart Study." *Circulation,* Vol. 67, No. 5, May 1983.

Hull, Elaine M., et al. "Aerobic Fitness Affects Cardiovascular Catecholamine Responses to Stressors." *Psychophysiology,* Vol. 21, No. 3, May 1984.

Hulley, Stephen B., M.D., et al. "Epidemiology as a Guide to Clinical Decisions."

Hurley, Ben F., Ph.D., et al. "High-Density Lipoprotein Cholesterol in Body-builders Versus Powerlifters." *Journal of the American Medical Association*, Vol. 252, No. 4, July 27, 1984.

Kannel, William B., M.D., and Lerner, Debra J., M.S. "Present Status of Risk Factors for Atherosclerosis." *Medical Times*, Vol. 112, No. 9, September 1984.

"Lowering Cholesterol Reduces the Risk of Heart Attack." *Internal Medicine Alert*, Vol. 6, No. 2, January 30, 1984.

Mahler, Donald A., M.D., et al. "Mechanical and Physiological Evaluation of Exercise Performance in Elite National Rowers." *Journal of the American Medical Association*, Vol. 252, No. 4, July 27, 1984.

Moser, Marvin, M.D. "High Blood Pressure and What You Can Do About It." The Benjamin Company, Inc., August 1983.

"Multiple Risk Factor Intervention Trial." *Journal of the American Medical Association*, Vol. 248, No. 12, September 24, 1982.

New York State Journal of Medicine, Vol. 83, No. 13, December 1983. Entire volume.

"Oral Contraceptives and the Risk of Cardiovascular Disease." *The Medical Letter*, Vol. 25, July 22, 1983.

Ornish, Dean, M.D., et al. "Effects of Stress Management Training and Dietary Changes in Treating Ischemic Heart Disease." *Journal of the American Medical Association*, Vol. 249, No. 1, January 7, 1983.

Paffenbarger, Ralph S., Jr., M.D., et al. "A Natural History of Athleticism and Cardiovascular Health." *Journal of the American Medical Association*, Vol. 252, No. 4, July 27, 1984.

Page, Lot B., M.D., et al. "Antecedents of Cardiovascular Disease in Six Solomon Islands Societies." *Circulation*, Vol. 49, June 1974.

Pedersen, Oluf, M.D., et al. "Increased Insulin Receptors After Exercise in Patients with Insulin-Dependent Diabetes Mellitus." *New England Journal of Medicine*, April 17, 1980.

Perspectives in Lipid Disorders, Vol. 1, No. 1, June 1983. Entire volume.

Roen, Paul B., M.D. "The Evening Meal and Atherosclerosis." *Journal of the American Geriatrics Society*, 1978.

Rogers, Robert L., M.A., et al. "Cigarette Smoking Decreases Cerebral Blood Flow Suggesting Increased Risk for Stroke." *Journal of the American Medical Association*, Vol. 250, No. 20, November 25, 1983.

Schoenberger, James A., M.D. "The Downward Trend in Cardiovascular Mortality: Challenge and Opportunity for the Practitioner." Editorials, *Journal of the American Medical Association*, Vol. 247, No. 6, February 12, 1982.

Shekelle, Richard B., Ph.D., et al. "Diet, Serum Cholesterol, and Death from Coronary Heart Disease." *New England Journal of Medicine*, Vol. 304, No. 2, January 8, 1981.

The Decline in Coronary Heart Disease Mortality—The Role of Cholesterol Change? Proceedings of a symposium held in Anaheim, California, November 13, 1983, in cooperation with the College of Physicians and Surgeons of Columbia University.

"The Effect of Treatment on Mortality in 'Mild' Hypertension." *New England Journal of Medicine*, October 14, 1982.

Thelle, Dag S., M.D., et al. "The Tromso Heart Study." *New England Journal of Medicine*, Vol. 308, No. 24, June 16, 1983.

"Treatment of Hypertriglyceridemia." *Journal of the American Medical Association*, Vol. 251, No. 9, March 2, 1984.

" 'Type A' Personalities in Men 'Mellowed' by Beta-Blockers." *Journal of the American Medical Association*, Vol. 247, No. 20, May 28, 1982.

Vander, Lauren B., M.S., et al. "Physiological Profile of National-Class National Collegiate Athletic Association Fencers." *Journal of the American Medical Association*, Vol. 252, No. 4, July 27, 1984.

White, Philip L., and Mondeika, Therese. *Diet and Exercise: Synergism in Health Maintenance.* Chicago: American Medical Association, 1982.

Williams, Paul T., et al. "The Effects of Running Mileage and Duration on Plasma Lipoprotein Levels." *Journal of the American Medical Association*, Vol. 247, No. 19, May 21, 1982.

Williams, R. Sanders, M.D., et al. "Physical Conditioning Augments the Fibrinolytic Response to Venous Occlusion in Healthy Adults." *New England Journal of Medicine*, Vol. 302, No. 18, May 1, 1980.

Wood, Dr. Peter D. "Running Away from Heart Disease." *Runner's World*, July 1979.

Zilversmit, Donald B., Ph.D., et al. "Diet and Cardiovascular Disease." *Professional Perspectives*, Division of Nutritional Sciences, Cornell University, June 1984.

Chapter Five

Blair, Steven N., PED, et al. "Improving Physical Fitness by Exercise Training Programs." *Southern Medical Journal*, Vol. 73, No. 12, December 1980.

Borg, G. "A Category Scale with Ratio Properties for Intermodal and Interindividual Comparisons." *Psychophysical Judgment and the Process of Perception*, Geissler, H. G., and Petzold, P., eds. Berlin: VEB Deutscher Verlag der Wissenschaften, 1982.

————. "Psychophysical Bases of Perceived Exertion." *Medicine and Science in Sports and Exercise,* Vol. 14, No. 5, 1982.

————. "Some General Functions and Their Differential Use." *Progress in Ergometry: Quality Control and Test Criteria,* Fifth International Seminar on Ergometry, Lollgen, H., and Mellerowicz, H., eds. Berlin: Springer-Verlag, 1984.

Borg, Gunnar A. V., and Marks, Lawrence E. "Twelve Meanings of the Measure Constant in Psychophysical Power Functions." *Bulletin of the Psychonomic Society,* Vol. 21, No. 1, 1983.

Cooper, Kenneth H., M.D. *The Aerobics Program for Total Well-Being.* New York: M. Evans and Company, Inc., 1982.

Dimsdale, Joel E., M.D., et al. "Post-exercise Peril." *Journal of the American Medical Association,* Vol. 251, No. 5, Feb. 3, 1984.

Hage, Philip. "Perceived Exertion: One Measure of Exercise Intensity." *The Physician and Sportsmedicine,* Vol. 9, No. 9, September 1981.

Marks, Lawrence E., et al. "Individual differences in perceived exertion assessed by two new methods." *Perception & Psychophysics,* 34, 3, 1983.

Chapter Six

Bassett, David R., Jr., et al. "Energy Cost of Simulated Rowing Using a Wind-Resistance Device." *The Physician and Sportsmedicine,* Vol. 12, No. 8, August 1984.

Cooper, Kenneth H., M.D. "Alternative Ways to Exercise." *Aerobics,* Vol. 5, No. 10, October 1984.

Day, Nancy Raines. "Fitness." *Health Information Library,* Daly City, Calif.: Krames Communications, 1983.

Dimsdale, Joel E., M.D., et al. "Post-exercise Peril." *Journal of the American Medical Association,* Vol. 251, No. 5, Feb. 3, 1984.

The Exercise Standards Book. American Heart Association, September, 1978. Revised edition, June, 1979.

"Getting the Beat for a Great Workout." *USA Today,* September 20, 1984.

Gettman, Larry R., et al. "A Comparison of Combined Running and Weight Training with Circuit-Weight Training." *Medicine and Science in Sports and Exercise,* Vol. 14, No. 3, 1982.

Leon, Arthur S., M.D., et al. "Effects of a Vigorous Walking Program on Body Composition and Carbohydrate and Lipid Metabolism of Obese Young Men." *American Journal of Clinical Nutrition,* Vol. 32, September, 1979.

"Pedal Down the Path to Better Health." *USA Today,* September 21, 1984.

"Special Aerobic Dance Section." *Shape,* Vol. 4, September, 1984.

Chapter Seven

Bruce, Robert A., M.D., et al. "Value of Maximal Exercise Testing in Risk Assessment of Primary Coronary Heart Disease Events in Healthy Men." *American Journal of Cardiology,* Vol. 46, September 1980.

Chaitman, Bernard R., M.D., and Hanson, John S., M.D. "Comparative Sensitivity and Specificity of Exercise Electrocardiographic Lead Systems." *American Journal of Cardiology,* Vol. 47, June 1981.

Cohn, Peter F., M.D. "The Role of Noninvasive Cardiac Testing after an Uncomplicated Myocardial Infarction." *New England Journal of Medicine,* Vol. 309, No. 2, July 14, 1983.

Froelicher, V. F., et al. "Value of Exercise Testing for Screening Asymptomatic Men for Latent Coronary Artery Disease." *Progress in Cardiovascular Diseases,* Vol. 18, No. 4, January-February, 1976.

Giagnoni, Erminia, M.D., et al. "Prognostic Value of Exercise ECG Testing in Asymptomatic Normotensive Subjects." *New England Journal of Medicine,* Vol. 309, No. 18, November 3, 1983.

Kasch, Fred W., Ph.D. "The Validity of the Astrand and Sjostrand Submaximal Tests." *The Physician and Sportsmedicine,* Vol. 12, No. 8, August 1984.

Kennedy, Robert H., M.D., et al. "Cardiac-Catheterization and Cardiac-Surgical Facilities." *New England Journal of Medicine,* Vol. 307, No. 16, October 14, 1982.

Miller, Albert J., M.D., et al. "Treadmill Exercise Testing in Hypertensive Patients Treated With Hydrochlorothiazide and B-Blocking Drugs." *Journal of the American Medical Association,* Vol. 250, No. 1, July 1, 1983.

Mills, R. M., Jr., M.D., and Greenberg, J. M., M.D. "A Clinical Approach to Exercise Tolerance Testing in Coronary Artery Disease." *Clinical Cardiology,* Vol. 6, July 1983.

Morris, Stephen N., M.D., and McHenry, Paul L., M.D. "Role of Exercise Stress Testing in Healthy Subjects and Patients With Coronary Heart Disease." *American Journal of Cardiology,* Vol. 42, October 1978.

Piepgrass, Sterling R., et al. "Limitations of the Exercise Stress Test in the Detection of Coronary Artery Disease in Apparently Healthy Men." *Aviation, Space, and Environmental Medicine,* April 1982.

Rozanski, Alan, M.D., et al. "The Declining Specificity of Exercise Radionuclide Ventriculography." *New England Journal of Medicine,* Vol. 309, No. 9, September 1, 1983.

Stone, Peter H., M.D. "Exercise Testing in Perspective." *Cardiac Rehabilitation,* Vol. 11, No. 4, Winter 1980.

Van Tellingen, Chris, et al. "On the Clinical Value of Conventional and New Exercise Electrocardiographic Criteria: A Comparative Study." *International Journal of Cardiology,* 1984.

Chapter Eight

Vega, Gloria Lena, and Grundy, Scott M. "Comparison of Apolipoprotein B to Cholesterol in Low Density Lipoproteins of Patients with Coronary Heart Disease." *Journal of Lipid Research,* Vol. 25, 1984.

Chapter Nine

"As Runners Extend Distances, Percent Reporting They Jog Levels Off; Half of Americans Exercise Regularly." *The Gallup Report,* No. 209, February 1983.

Billman, George E., Ph.D., et al. "The Effects of Daily Exercise on Susceptibility to Sudden Cardiac Death." *Circulation,* Vol. 69, No. 6, June 1984.

Cooper, Lt. Col. Kenneth H., MC, USAF, "Guidelines in the Management of the Exercising Patient." *Journal of the American Medical Association,* Vol. 211, No. 10, March 9, 1970.

"Does Vigorous Exercise Protect Against or Provoke Sudden Cardiac Death?—The Answer Is Probably Both." *Internal Medicine Alert,* Vol. 6, No. 19, October 15, 1984.

"Exercise Benefits Older People, Report Says." *American Medical News,* August 10, 1984.

"Exercise for Bypass Patients." New York: CJ Publishing Company.

Froelicher, Victor, M.D., et al. "A Randomized Trial of Exercise Training in Patients With Coronary Heart Disease." *Journal of the American Medical Association,* Vol. 252, No. 10, September 14, 1984.

Gotto, Antonio M., Jr., M.D. "Symposium on High Density Lipoproteins and Coronary Artery Disease: Effects of Diet, Exercise, and Pharmacologic Intervention." *American Journal of Cardiology,* Vol. 52, No. 4, August 22, 1983.

Grundy, Scott M., M.D. "Can Modification of Risk Factors Reduce Coronary Heart Disease?" *Controversies in Coronary Artery Disease,* 1982.

Hagan, R. D., Ph.D., and Gettman, L. R., Ph.D. "Maximal Aerobic Power, Body Fat, and Serum Lipoproteins in Male Distance Runners." *Journal of Cardiac Rehabilitation*, Vol. 3, No. 5, May 1983.

"Hope Grows for Vigorous Old Age." *The New York Times*, October 2, 1984.

Kramsch, Dieter M., M.D., et al. "Reduction of Coronary Atherosclerosis by Moderate Conditioning Exercise In Monkeys on an Atherogenic Diet." *New England Journal of Medicine*, Vol. 305, No. 25, December 17, 1981.

Myerburg, Robert J., M.D., et al. "Survivors of Prehospital Cardiac Arrest." *Journal of the American Medical Association*, Vol. 247, No. 10, March 12, 1982.

"Myocardial Infarction and Mortality in the Coronary Artery Surgery Study (CASS) Randomized Trial." *New England Journal of Medicine*, Vol. 310, No. 12, March 22, 1984.

"Regression of Atherosclerosis: Preliminary but Encouraging News." Medical News, *Journal of the American Medical Association*, Vol. 246, No. 20, November 20, 1981.

Seals, Douglas R., Ph.D., et al. "Effects of Endurance Training on Glucose Tolerance and Plasma Lipid Levels in Older Men and Women." *Journal of the American Medical Association*, Vol. 252, No. 5, August 3, 1984.

Simon, Harvey B., M.D. "The Immunology of Exercise." *Journal of the American Medical Association*, Vol. 252, No. 19, November 16, 1984.

Sports Injuries: An Aid to Prevention and Treatment, funded by Bufferin for the American College of Sports Medicine, the American Orthopedic Society for Sports Medicine and the Sports Medicine Committee of the United States Tennis Association.

"Sudden Cardiac Death: Are Runners at Risk?" New York: CJ Publishing Company.

Thoresen, Carl E., et al. "The Recurrent Coronary Prevention Project: Some Preliminary Findings." *Acta Med Scan* (Suppl.) 660: 172–192, 1982.

The Veterans Administration Coronary Artery Bypass Surgery Cooperative Study Group. "Eleven-Year Survival in the Veterans Administration Randomized Trial of Coronary Bypass Surgery For Stable Angina." *New England Journal of Medicine*, Vol. 311, No. 21, November 22, 1984.

Wood, Peter D., et al. "Increased Exercise Level and Plasma Lipoprotein Concentrations: A One-Year, Randomized, Controlled Study in Sedentary, Middle-Aged Men." *Metabolism*, Vol. 32, No. 1, January 1983.

Wood, Peter D., and Haskell, William L. "The Effect of Exercise on Plasma High-Density Lipoproteins." *Lipids*, Vol. 14, No. 4, 1979.

Chapter Ten

"Cardiovascular Death Toll Decreases Sharply." *American Medical News,* February 19, 1982.

"Cut Your Insurance Bill." *USA Today,* November 10, 1983.

Dismuke, S. Edwards, M.D., and Miller, Stephen T., M.D. "Why Not Share the Secrets of Good Health?" *Journal of the American Medical Association,* Vol. 249, No. 23, June 17, 1983.

"Expert: Many Hospitals to Close." *Dallas Times-Herald,* April 18, 1982.

Golden, Patricia M., and Wilson, Ronald W. *Prevention Profile: Excerpted From Health, United States 1983,* National Center for Health Statistics, Public Health Service, U.S. Department of Health and Human Services.

"Has the Fitness Boom Gone Bust?" *Athletic Purchasing and Facilities,* July 1983.

"Health Care Soon Up to $1 Billion a Day." *American Medical News.* (Undated)

"Health Organizations Square Off Against Tobacco Defense Ads." *American Medical News,* March 2, 1984.

"Hospitals Try Varied Tactics in Battle for Patient Dollars." *American Medical News,* August 13, 1982.

"Indonesians Get in Shape." *Honolulu Advertiser,* March 13, 1984.

McGehee, Pittman. Sunday Program, Christ Church Cathedral, Houston, Texas, July 29, 1984.

"Non-smoking Discount Offered." *American Medical News,* January 13, 1984.

"Reasons for Heart Disease Death Rate Decline Sought." *Valley Morning Star,* January 6, 1982.

Stokes, Joseph, III, M.D. "Why Not Rate Health and Life Insurance Premiums By Risks?" *New England Journal of Medicine,* Vol. 308, No. 7, February 17, 1983.

"Surgeon General Heralds Decline." *Dallas Times-Herald,* May 28, 1980.

"We're Smoking Less: It's Too Expensive." *USA Today,* March 9, 1984.

GLOSSARY

aerobic   living or exercising in air; a body which is in homeostatic balance, with the same amount of oxygen being used as is being taken in.

anaerobic   a bodily state where more oxygen is required than is being taken in; the usual result is exhaustion.

angina pectoris   chest pain caused by spasm of one of the coronary arteries or a deficiency of blood to the heart in some other way.

arteriosclerosis   clogging or blockage of the arteries with fatty deposits of cholesterol; hardening of the arteries.

ASH   asymmetric septal hypertrophy, which involves an unusual thickness of the wall separating the two lower chambers of the heart.

asymmetric   uneven.

atherosclerosis   same as arteriosclerosis.

Balke Protocol   a procedure for taking a treadmill stress test which utilizes a constant speed and progressive incline, until the twenty-fifth minute.

beta-blocker   drug commonly used to treat hypertension and other heart-related problems.

biventricular hypertrophy   excessively large lower chambers of the heart.

233

bradycardia   abnormally slow heart rate.

Bruce Protocol   a procedure for taking a treadmill stress test which increases both speed and incline every three minutes. To convert the time on the Bruce Protocol to the Balke, multiply the time in minutes by 1.75.

bypass operation   surgery on the heart that involves grafting in vessels which "bypass" coronary arteries that are clogged by arteriosclerosis.

cardiac   related to the heart.

cardiac arrhythmia   irregular heart beat.

cardiovascular   relating to the blood vessels and the heart.

cholesterol   a fatty substance in the blood that is associated with arteriosclerosis, or hardening of the arteries.

click   extra sound made by the heart, often because of a "floppy" mitral valve.

congenital   existing at birth.

control group   a group of individuals in a scientific test against whom other groups are tested. Typically, the "controls" remain the same before, during, and after the test. That is, there is no medical intervention to try to change their status.

cool-down   the all-important final phase of physical exercise during which the rate of bodily activity is gradually decreased.

coronary arteries   arteries supplying the heart muscle.

coronary arteriography   the procedure of inserting a tube into an artery, depositing a dye into the coronary arteries, and then taking an X-ray of the degree of clogging of those arteries. Same as coronary angiography.

echocardiogram   a "picture" of the heart taken by bouncing sound waves off the heart muscle.

electrocardiogram   tracings on graph paper that record the electrical impulses of the heart; also referred to as an ECG or EKG.

electrode   a rubber patch with wires leading to an electrocardiograph.

endorphin   morphine-like substance released by the pituitary gland in a variety of situations, including vigorous exercise.

epinephrine   a natural stimulant produced by the adrenal glands; also called "adrenaline."

ergometer   an apparatus used to measure the work performed by a group of muscles.

false negative   a stress test result indicating there is no disease or abnormality when there actually is.

false positive a stress test result indicating the presence of disease or other abnormality when actually nothing is wrong with the individual.

high density lipoprotein a component of blood cholesterol which is thought to limit or reduce the build-up of fatty deposits or arteriosclerosis in the blood vessels. Also referred to as HDL.

Holter monitoring a procedure involving the recording on magnetic tape of the heart's electrical signals as they are emitted during an ECG over a period of twenty-four hours. Then, the signals are replayed and scanned to detect slight changes that might go unnoticed in an ordinary electrocardiogram.

hypertrophic cardiomyopathy an abnormally enlarged heart with thickened heart tissue; also called HCM.

hypertrophy enlargement of an organ, such as the heart.

IHSS idiopathic hypertrophic subaortic stenosis. This refers to a thickening in the ventricular septum directly below the aortic valve, which may result in obstruction to the outflow of blood from the heart, particularly during exercise. It is also called hypertrophic cardiomyopathy.

ischemia lack of blood supply to an organ because of a deficiency in blood flow through an artery.

lead a field of electrical activity emitted by the action of the heart muscle and recorded by an electrocardiogram.

lipid fatty substance in the blood.

low density lipoprotein a component of blood cholesterol which is thought to promote the build-up of fatty deposits or arteriosclerosis in the blood vessels. Also referred to as LDL.

Masters two-step a stress test that requires the individual being tested to step up and down on a raised platform.

MUGA scan an acronym standing for Multiple-Gated Acquisition. This is a specialized test that involves techniques of nuclear medicine that are still being developed.

murmur swishing sound caused as the blood moves in an unusual way through the various chambers and valves of the heart.

myocardial infarction heart attack.

myocarditis inflammation of the heart muscle.

negative treadmill stress test a normal test that has no abnormal patient or ECG response.

norepinephrine natural stimulant produced by the adrenal glands.

obesity percentage of body fat; *not* just the amount a person is overweight according to weight and body-type tables.

PMHR predicted maximum heart rate.

positive treadmill stress test an abnormal test due either to the patient response or to an abnormal electrocardiogram.

predicted maximum heart rate the maximum expected rate that a person's heart can reach during vigorous exercise, given the person's age and state of fitness.

prolapsed mitral valve an abnormal condition of a heart valve, usually affecting young women. Also known as Barlow's Syndrome and the Mid-Systolic Click Syndrome.

risk factor a feature in a person's heredity, background, or present lifestyle that increases the likelihood of developing coronary heart disease.

sensitivity the degree of true readings in a stress test.

septum a wall, such as that separating the two ventricles of the heart.

serial change a change for the worse in a treadmill stress test when all previous tests have been normal.

S-T segment the last line of one of the heart's contractions during exercise, as traced on an electrocardiogram. This line is considered of key importance in determining the presence of heart disease.

sudden death death occurring within six hours of the onset of symptoms.

target heart rate the heart rate during exercise at which the greatest training benefit occurs, usually 65 to 85 percent of predicted maximum heart rate.

thallium scan a test in which a radioisotopic material is injected into a vein and then scanned with a special instrument in an effort to diagnose heart disease.

treadmill stress test (TMST) a procedure to determine a person's degree of fitness and cardiovascular health. In a properly conducted stress test, the patient walks to exhaustion on a treadmill with a moving, motorized belt.

triglycerides fatty substances in the blood that are the major constituents of very low density lipoprotein (VLDL).

ventricles the two lower heart chambers.

ventricular fibrillation irregular fluttering of the heart, which, if uninterrupted, often results in death.

ventricular septum the wall that separates the two lower heart chambers.

ventricular tachycardia excessively high heart rate.

INDEX